Trends in Wound Care

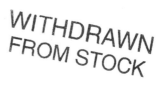
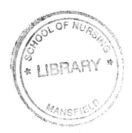

Trends in Wound Care
BJN monograph

edited by
Richard White

Quay Books

Mark Allen
Publishing Ltd

100312 2117

Quay Books Division, Mark Allen Publishing Limited,
Jesses Farm, Snow Hill, Dinton, Wiltshire, SP3 5HN

British Library Cataloguing-in-Publication Data
A catalogue record is available for this book

© Mark Allen Publishing Ltd 2002
ISBN 1 85642 170 8

Printed in the UK by The Bath Press, Bath

Contents

Section IV: Practice

List of contributors

Kate Ballard is Clinical Nurse Specialist, Tissue Viability, Tissue Viability Unit, Guy's Nuffield House, London.

Helena Baxter is Education and Practice Project Officer, Hinchinbrook Hospital, Huntingdon.

Rose Cooper is Principal Lecturer in Microbiology, School of Applied Sciences, University of Wales Institute, Cardiff.

Fiona Culley is an Independent Nurse Advisor, St Alban's, Hertfordshire.

Lorraine Foster is Review Manager, Commission for Health Improvement, Finsbury Tower, London EC1Y 8TG.

Janet L Hadcock is Research Practitioner/Expert Nurse, Intensive Care Unit, Salford Royal Hospitals NHS Trust, Hope Hospital, Salford, Manchester.

Andrew Kingsley is Clinical Nurse Specialist, Tissue Viability and Infection Control, North Devon District Hospital, Barnstaple.

Peter Moore is Consultant General Surgeon, Northern Lincolnshire and Goole NHS Trust.

Lynn Parker is Infection Control Nurse, Scunthorpe General Hospital, Cliff Gardens, Scunthorpe.

Linda Russell is Tissue Viability Nurse Specialist, Queen's Hospital, Burton Hospitals NHS Trust, Burton-on-Trent, Staffordshire.

Peter Vowden is Consultant Vascular Surgeon, Bradford Royal Infirmary.

Kathryn Vowden is Clinical Nurse Specialist, Department of Vascular Surgery, Bradford Royal Infirmary and Lecturer, University of Bradford.

Richard White is a Clinical Research Consultant and Medical Writer, Highbury House, Whitstone, Holsworthy, Cornwall.

Trudie Young is Lecturer in Tissue Viability, School of Nursing, Glan Clwyd Hospital, Bodelwyddan, Denbighshire, North Wales.

Foreword

Some colleagues may say 'not another book on wounds' but I would urge you to recognise the value of the information contained within this book. At a time when there is increasing professional interest in the subject, an explosion of new therapies and a demand for evidence-based practice there is an increasing need for comprehensive sources of information.

The monograph series of the *British Journal of Nursing* have dealt with a wide range of essential subjects in current day practice, but this volume on wound care provides in many ways a novel and unique approach to this important, wide-ranging and often confusing subject. Under the editorship of Dr Richard White and his team of experts in the field you have a comprehensive review of a number of essential aspects of wound care. The four sections deal not only with theory specific to wound types but also practice issues.

Provision of appropriate standards of care to patients requires a good understanding of the basics of wound healing and controversies surrounding aspects of infection are also discussed. The practical advice contained in the section on chronic wounds helps clinicians who are working at the 'coal face' to offer excellent care to their patients. The section on acute wounds and aspects of clinical practice in an accident and emergency department, in addition to wound care in an ICU, are often forgotten in other books on this subject but affect a large number of patients and healthcare professionals. The section on practice deals with challenging issues associated with documentation and classification of wounds in addition to the important but under-researched area of nutrition.

There is a momentum currently pushing wound care both upwards in the minds of healthcare staff and forwards in the development of an evidence-based important clinical subject. The need for more research, education and information in this area is both urgent and on a large scale. This book provides a novel and practical approach that will assist clinicians both in their thinking and also in improving the care of their patients. Read, digest and enjoy.

Keith Harding
February, 2002

Introduction

In recent years the increased focus on research in wound care, both clinical and scientific, has resulted in a vast increase of reports in the published literature. To accommodate this, several new journals have appeared, each aimed at a specific aspect of wound care. Regular readers of the *British Journal of Nursing* will also have noticed an increasing number of wound-related articles, as well as the new 'Tissue Viability' supplement. This reflects the clinical, scientific and financial importance of wound care to the nursing profession.

This compilation of selected articles from established authorities in their respective areas, is sourced from the *British Journal of Nursing* 1999–2001 and subsequently expanded, amended and updated by the authors. It is intended to present a coherent update on significant developments in the field of wound care nursing. The four sections cover basic wound healing physiology, current diagnostic and treatment standards, progress in acute and chronic wound management, and, implications for clinical practice.

The editor and the publishers intend that this be the first volume in a regular, annual sequence textbook dedicated to providing the nursing profession with a concise 'state of the art' manual.

Richard White
Whitstone
February, 2002

Acknowledgements

My thanks to all the contributors of this monograph for their invaluable support, to Binkie Mais of Quay Books for her help in its preparation, and also to Keith Harding for his foreword.

Section I:
Basics

1

Understanding physiology of wound healing and how dressings help

Linda Russell

One of the most fascinating features of the human body is its ability to repair damaged tissue. When the skin is injured a complex process occurs. The natural healing process can be divided into four distinct stages: inflammatory, granulation, epithelialisation and maturation. This process can take up to two years. Brunner and Suddarth (1992) classified wound healing into three stages: primary; secondary; and tertiary. Many factors affect how long a wound will take to heal, eg. concurrent illness, nutritional status and the dressing used. A holistic approach to wound care is the key, and if all the factors are not addressed then wound healing will not prevail.

A complex set of events occurs upon injury to the skin, which appear to be relatively simple but, in fact, are exceptionally complicated giving rise to physical and chemical reactions and cellular episodes. Flanagan (1996) states that 'wound healing can be defined as the physiological process by which the body replaces and restores the function of damaged tissue'. Despite the large amount of research that has been undertaken in this field, there are still areas which are not properly understood.

Wound healing

The natural healing process can be divided into four stages: inflammatory, granulation, epithelialisation and maturation.

Inflammatory process: The inflammatory process is a 'biological emergency' response with a latent stage of about twelve hours before any obvious healing begins (Silver, 1994). However, the activity before this is very concentrated with many complex chemical events occurring. Once an injury has been sustained by the body, platelets are released from the blood vessel, which initiate haemostasis coagulation of blood leaking from damaged, inflamed, dilated blood vessels (Kerstein, 1997). At the same time a biochemical cascade occurs that liberates thrombokinase and this is converted to thrombin. The clots from fibrinogen are converted to fibrin, which covers the wound, and brings the wound edges together. Neutrophils (white blood cells) are attracted into the wound within hours of injury. A series of elaborate messages are initiated which cause blood cells to proceed to the site of the injury bringing extra oxygen supplies to the wound and phagocytes to clear tissue debris.

Also, there is release of growth factors, several cytokines which include regulatory peptides and glycopeptides (Hopkinson, 1992). On injury, damaged cells release inflammatory mediators such as prostaglandins and histamine from mast cells. Serotonin may also be released from the basophils (also known as mast cells) that results in vasodilatation from the existing blood vessels and increased cell permeability for the neutrophils and monocytes and other white blood cells (T and B lymphocytes), thus improving the blood supply to the wound.

The reason for this increased blood supply is to remove the toxins and dead cells (Tortora and Anagnostakos, 1987). Wound cleansing is commenced by the macrophages by the process of phagocytosis. Throughout the healing process macrophages are circulating and produce chemical messages to initiate wound healing (Butterworth *et al*, 1992). Macrophages and neutrophils are essential for the transition from the inflammatory to proliferative phase of healing (Silver, 1992).

Macrophages arrive one to two days and digest the fibrin and provide the defence against infection. There are also growth factors that initiate formation of fibroblasts and structural protein, and collagen for angiogenesis — the next phase of wound healing (Kerstein, 1997; Morison *et al*, 1997). The interleukins — cytokines — are involved in inflammation and wound healing and affect local tissue by increasing tissue adhesion and attraction of T and B lymphocytes to the site of injury.

Erythema occurs as a result of the blood vessels expanding and increasing blood supply. The endothelial cells become more permeable and this fluid may leak into the surrounding area (extravasation). The combination of these processes results in oedema, which may last for up to three days after injury (Tortora and Anagnostakos, 1987; Collier, 1996). The clinical signs of inflammation were first outlined by Celsus in AD 100 'as rubor (redness), calor (heat), dolor (pain), and oedema (swelling)' (Dealey, 1994).

The literature demonstrates that the regeneration phase ranges from three to twenty-four days and can be divided into two sections: granulation and epithelialisation.

Granulation: This occurs in deep dermal wounds (Ghen and Hutchinson, 1998). Macrophages signal to the dermal fibroblasts to lay fibrils of reticulin across the wound. This is later converted to collagen. The next stage is commencement of angiogenesis. New granulation tissue is very vascular due to capillary loops, which give the tissue its classic red appearance. New tissue is composed of macrophages, fibroblasts, capillary buds and loops in a matrix of fibronectin, collagen and hyaluronic acid (Dealey, 1994). Prolonged starvation of oxygen supply will reduce the mobility of the fibroblasts and delay healing (*Figure 1.1*). Angiogenesis is the growth of new blood vessels which are activated by tissue hypoxia from the disruption of the blood at the time of injury (Flanagan, 1997a).

As new tissue is laid down, the wound edges contract, then the growth factors interact with the mediator cells that cause the myosin bundles to approximate the wound edges. This occurs on the fifth or sixth day after injury. Flanagan (1997a) suggests that wound contraction only occurs when the wound bed consists of healthy granulation tissue: '... this explains why no reduction in the wound size occurs until the base of the wound has been shallowed out' (Flanagan, 1997b). Large deep wounds will take a considerable time to contract and demonstrate healing. Contraction could be responsible for 40–80% of wound closure (*Figure 1.2*) (Irvin and Challopadhyay, 1978). If the inflammatory progress is prolonged at this stage, over granulation can occur with hypertrophic scarring.

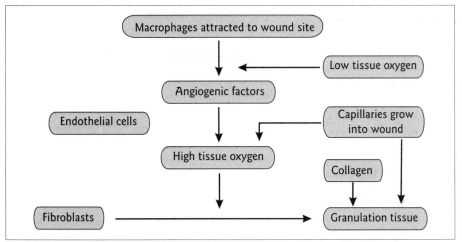

Figure 1.1: Healing process from injury to granulation. Adapted from Davis *et al*, 1992

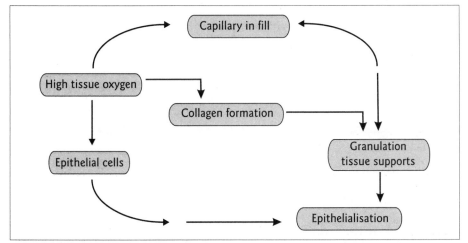

Figure 1.2: The process of healing for full-thickness injury through to epithelialisation. Adapted from Davis *et al*, 1992

Epithelialisation: This is the final stage of wound healing in shallow superficial wounds above the dermis and occurs quicker in small wounds than in wounds healed by secondary intention. Following the high activity from the growth factors cocktail, macrophages and fibroblasts continue to produce new dermis rich in collagen, hyaluronan, fibronectin, keratinocytes, hair follicles and sebaceous glands. Epithelialisation is achieved by squamous cells migrating across the wound surface until the deficit is resolved (Dealey, 1994; Chen and Hutchinson, 1998). This very delicate tissue survival is dependent on a moist environment (Winter, 1962). The new epithelial tissue is pinkish-white, which gives a translucent appearance, and is seen in granulating wounds (Flanagan, 1997a).

Remodelling/maturation: This stage can take from twenty-four days to two years to complete. Tissue which has been deposited over the wound is fragile and therefore needs to be strengthened by more robust collagen and extracellular matrix. The main components responsible for this stage are fibroblasts and macrophages. New tissue will only gain up to 80% of its strength before the biological emergency (*Figure 1.3*) (Chen and Hutchinson, 1998). This is the stage where the healing process switches off, vascularisation to the wound decreases, fibroblasts decrease, collagen matures and the appearance of granulation tissue changes from red to white. If a scab has been present, this will detach itself leaving new tissue underneath (Collier, 1996).

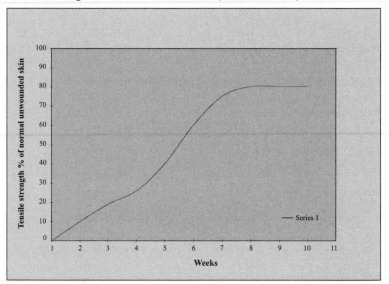

Figure 1.3: The tensile strength of a wound during the healing process. Adapted from Davis *et al*, 1992

Definitions of healing intention

Brunner and Suddarth (1992) classified wound healing into three stages: primary, secondary and tertiary.

Primary intention: These wounds are usually superficial breaks in the skin through trauma or surgical procedures. Skin edges are brought together with sutures, staples or glue to enable a very fine scar to form. Primary healing is often rapid with minimal scarring (Collier, 1996).

Secondary intention: Wounds healed by secondary intention extend into the dermis or deeper layers and the defects fill slowly with new cells. These wounds may be chronic and long-standing, eg. leg ulcers or pressure sores. They may also become infected. A holistic view needs to be taken for the management of this type of patient.

Tertiary intention: These occur when the wound has broken down following a surgical procedure. Often these wounds are infected and require surgical intervention to identify and remove the cause that may be either haematoma or large collections of pus, which may also cause wound dehiscence.

Factors that can delay wound healing

Moist wound healing

Gilge (1948) studied the effect of a moist environment on venous ulcers healed under Unna's boot and demonstrated quicker healing rates. The 'optimum environment for the natural wound healing process to be activated is warm, moist and non-toxic' (Winter, 1975). Drying the wound will cause the healing process to cease. Eaglstein (1985) demonstrated that when wounds were left exposed to the air or dressed with traditional gauze dressing, which tends to lead to wound drying, the healing rate decreases by 40% when compared to a moist wound where epidermal resurfacing took place rapidly.

Field and Kerstein (1994) suggested that there are distinct advantages of moist wound healing for the patient. There is less pain because the wound is immersed in the natural body fluids and fewer infections will result, as dry eschar may harbour micro-organisms. There is also reduced trauma when dressings are changed as they will not adhere to a moist wound, with less chance of micro-organism transmission and less airborne dispersal of dried fragments of wound tissue. Autolytic debridement occurs more effectively in a moist environment and the majority of dressings require water for the hydrolysis of proteins.

Wound exudate

Multiple components constitute wound exudate, both in terms of the nature and volume of exudate, eg. blood vessels, growth factors and wound debris, dead cells, extracellular matrix and micro-organisms (Chen and Hutchinson, 1998). Exudate also contains red blood cells and platelets that have been filtered out as the fluid passes through capillary walls into the surrounding wound (Thomas, 1997). A sudden increase in exudate may be an early indication that an infection is imminent. The production of wound exudate is dependent on many factors, eg. whether the wound is chronic or acute. The exudate from acute wounds is abundant in growth factors which have been shown to promote wound healing (Madden and Finkelstein, 1989; Chen and Rogers, 1992; Ono and Gunji, 1994).

Very little is known on the amount of exudate produced from different wounds. Thomas (1997) and Lamke and Nilsson (1997) demonstrated that burns and leg ulcers can produce in excess of $5000g/m^2$/day. It is generally agreed that a decrease in the amount of exudate means that wound healing is occurring.

Thomas (1997) indicates that even highly experienced nurses are unable to classify wounds accurately according to the amount of exudate production. He studied 10 leg ulcers and measured the exudate from each patient which ranged from 0.4 to $1.2g/cm^2$/24 hours ($4000–12000g/1m^2$/day). He discovered that interpatient variation did not correlate with the subjective impressions of the investigators. Therefore, nurses should closely monitor exudate output and, where possible, document how much fluid has been lost from the wound, instead of just classifying exudate as light, moderate or heavy and assuming that everybody's perceptions are the same.

However, chronic wounds tend to contain large amounts of degrading tissue and this can actually delay wound healing (Grinnell and Zhu, 1994, 1996; Rogers *et al*, 1995; Wysocki, 1996). Infected wounds have a different exudate and encompass degrading tissue as well as bacterial toxins, which may indirectly delay wound healing. Excessive exudate results in skin maceration, resulting in further tissue damage around the wound which needs to be taken into account when selecting a dressing.

Age and the effects on wound healing

Ferguson (1993) stated that:

We are ignorant of the basic scientific processes underlying wound healing, particularly in the elderly... this ignorance and resulting deficiencies in clinical management mean that the majority of wounds are maintained by nursing and medical care, not cured.

Foetal wound healing has demonstrated that full-thickness wounds can heal without scarring and is dependent on the intrauterine development (Adzick *et al*, 1985). Children have a more vigorous healing rate, from the age of one to three years the dermis increases in thickness and from the age of four to seven years the dermis doubles in thickness (Morison *et al*, 1997).

Associated with ageing are the physiological changes in the body, and these can lead to a predisposition to injury and decreased efficiency of wound healing mechanisms (Morison *et al*, 1997). However, our bodies age at different rates and over the age of thirty years a significant decline may occur in some systems, such as the cardiac and immune systems, which in part can contribute to longer healing times. Replacement of epidermal cells, inflammatory response, sensory perception and barrier function all decrease through the ageing process. Arterial and venous disease can delay wound healing and are a common problem in the elderly population. The effect of ageing is often compounded by concurrent illness and malnutrition. Long-standing chronic illness is known to impair appetite, as may drugs, anxiety, depression and radiotherapy (Bond, 1998).

Wounds in elderly people do, however, heal with good effect in most instances but it takes longer (Davis *et al*, 1992). Assessment of the patient is very important and identifying the risk factors to their vulnerability is vital with the use of risk assessment tools used for pressure sores.

Temperature of the wound

The ideal wound temperature has been identified as 37°C. A reduced temperature may inhibit the activity of cells involved with the healing process (Lock, 1980). The optimum environment is required for natural enzymes that are secreted by inflammatory cells to continue the sequence of wound healing. Modern dressings are designed to maintain this optimum temperature of 37°C. If the wound temperature falls below 28°C then leukocyte activity can stop, particularly if dressings are removed for ward rounds. Wounds should be covered with sterile cling film to maintain temperature and moisture. The reduction in wound temperature can take several hours to recover to full mitotic activity (Lock, 1980).

Wound dressings

A huge array of dressing products are currently on the market which can be confusing to the nurse trying to decide which product to use. The demand for wound care products is growing rapidly due to demographic and technological changes (Roberts, 1998). Numerous clinical trials are now performed in order to produce clinical evidence for products. The evidence should be subjected to rigorous evaluation, including cost implications of the treatment and the healing time to the end point. Many of the current clinical trials do not address these problems.

A reason for the focus on increased efficacy of wound care products is that purchasers and the Government are concentrating on cost-effective care and measurable outcomes in treatment. Roberts (1998) suggests that cost-effective management of wounds is a complex matter and should not only concentrate on short-term healing costs, but also consider the long-term expenses. The total costs of dressings are hard to ascertain because not only do nurses apply dressings but they may also be applied by physiotherapists and chiropodists. Thus, the amount of inappropriate wound care that actually takes place is hard to detect. Professionals are now calling for clinical evidence that a product is cost-effective and promotes quick healing. Economic evaluation should consider:

- cost-minimisation: outcome (ie. healing) equal but price of products different
- cost-effectiveness: clinical benefit in better efficacy drives true cost benefit
- cost-utility: links cost in conjunction with health gain
- cost-benefit: attempts to value all costs and consequences in same units.

The history of modern-day dressings is fascinating. In the early 1970s there were a limited number of dressings available, which were mainly traditional, eg. gauze. One reason for the change of dressing products in the 1980s was the discovery that new blood vessels grow from zones rich in oxygen towards those with less oxygen (Knighton *et al*, 1983). Lydon and Hutchinson (1989) demonstrated that angiogenesis occurs more rapidly in wounds covered with hydrocolloids.

At the same time that hydrocolloids were being developed, foam dressings were also being launched. The 1980s saw the introduction of hydrocolloids into routine use which encouraged moist wound healing. Further competition between manufacturers led to the subsequent introduction of hydrogels and alginates. Technological developments have progressed to such an extent that skin replacement has now become easier. However, this is currently very expensive but cost will decrease as the demand increases.

Economics of dressings

The amount of money spent in 1999 in the UK on modern wound care products was £80 000 000 (International Monetary Fund [IMF] Data, 1999, personal communication). This can be apportioned into the hospital (£14 000 000) and community (£74 000 00). A further £15 000 000 in the community and £6 000 000 in hospitals is spent on traditional dressings (IMF Data, 1999). Dealey (1994) states that second-generation dressings are considerably more expensive than the traditional dressings they have replaced. The cost of gauze is only a few pence and products that cost £1–2 per dressing appear very expensive (*Table 1.1*). However, with these new dressings the wounds will not need daily changes and this may well promote quicker wound healing and save nursing time (Dealey, 1994).

Table 1.1: Cost comparison of gauze daily dressing to one modern application once a week		
	Traditional gauze twice daily dressings	Modern dressing Aquacel and Combiderm
Cost of dressing packs	£0.60 x 2*	£0.60*
Cavity dressing	£20.50*	£7.65* Aquacel ribbon x 3
Secondary dressing	£6.00*	£6.96* Combiderm x 4
Normal saline	£1.50*	£1.50*
Tape	£1.63*	
Total	£30.83	£16.71

*These costs are average and do not include nursing time; adapted from Roberts and McLoughlin, 1997

Patient compliance with dressing products

With a vast choice of products on the market, patients' acceptability of the dressing should be taken into consideration. A dressing that allows the patient to undertake normal activity will result in high compliance with treatment. In particular, the use of modern wound dressings reduces the costs of nursing time and follow-up visits. Madden and Finkelstein (1989), Newmeth and Eaglstein (1991), and Heffernan and Martin (1994) have demonstrated that hydrocolloids constantly reduced pain on removal when compared to gauze. Furthermore, hydrocolloid products can be left in place for up to seven days (Siegal, 1996). Miller and Collier (1996) suggest that patient compliance will be enhanced when a dressing is chosen collectively with the patient.

Dressings

Having performed a holistic assessment of the wound, optimum surroundings need to be maintained to promote the natural wound healing process such as a warm, moist, non-toxic environment (Winter, 1975; Thomas, 1990). Thomas (1997) states that if these optimum conditions are met, the result is faster healing, less scar formation, fewer dressing changes, less pain and reduction in the infection rates. 'Wound healing is a continuum, and it is likely that the effect of dressings on one phase of the process influences events during the next phase' (Newmeth and Eaglstein, 1991).

Winter (1962) researched the theory that has formed the foundation of modern dressing development. He compared dry wounds and moist wounds and discovered that moist wounds granulated up to 40% faster than dry wounds. The benefits of moist healing are summarised in *Table 1.2*. A dressing, therefore, has to: maintain a moist, but not macerated, surface; allow gaseous exchange; prevent bacteria from entering the wound; allow removal of excess exudate; maintain the wound temperature at 37°C; ensure no trauma occurs on removal; and keep the wound at the ideal pH value.

A knowledgeable practitioner should have an understanding of not only the physiology of wound healing but also the dressing products they will employ to promote wound healing (Collier, 1996). In addition, Thomas (1997) states that a greater understanding is required of the properties and performance of individual wound care products, particularly in respect to fluid management characteristics.

Table 1.2: The benefits of moist wound healing	
Outcome or benefit	Possible explanation provided
Less reported benefit	Free nerve endings responsible for pain are bathed in physiological fluids
Fewer infections reported	Viable host defences, less dry dead tissue to harbour micro-organisms
Less re-injury on removal	Moist wound healing interface
Less risk of micro-organism transmission	Less airborne dispersal of micro-organisms on removal
Efficient autolytic debridement versus mechanical for traditional drying dressings	Enzymes require water for hydrolysis of proteins

Adapted from Field and Kerstein, 1994

Pain on dressing change

McCaffrey (1983) states: 'Pain is what the patient says it is and exists when he says it does.' Waugh (1990) states that social and cultural factors, personality and current psychological state influence pain perceptions. Morison (1992) suggests that a dressing chart should include a pain scale of 0–10. This would encourage the nurse to document the patient's perception of pain and the frequency. Factors which cause pain include inflammation, exposure to the air, pressure on local tissue or movement, dressing change, irritant chemicals, clinical infection and suture removal (Morison, 1992).

Pain and discomfort are often the body's warning bell, eg. a wound infection. At this stage a wound must be inspected and assessed (Davis *et al*, 1992). Where possible all the factors that contribute to pain need to be taken into consideration and the appropriate analgesia given before dressing change. The characteristics of dressing products are shown in *Table 1.3*.

Conclusion

It is essential to have good knowledge of anatomy and physiology of wound healing and factors that can affect the rate of healing. A holistic patient assessment needs to be made and all factors need to be considered and pieced together. If there are deficiencies they need to be identified and corrected where possible. Understanding of the dressing employed to manage a patient's wound is also very important, particularly with the huge array of products available on the market. More research needs to be undertaken in relation to the cost and efficacy of products and healing rates. Primarily, the nurse is in a pivotal position to help promote cost-effective wound healing.

Table 1.3: Characteristics of dressing products	
Film membranes	Permeable to water vapour and oxygen; impermeable to water and micro-organisms; provide a warm, moist environment; comfortable; convenient; permit constant observation
Foams	Provide thermal insulation; do not shed particles; maintain a moist environment; gas permeable; non-adherent; absorb significant amounts of exudate; easily removed
Hydrogels	Rehydrate wounds; debride and clean; painless to apply and remove; soothing
Hydrocolloids	Provide a warm, moist environment; impermeable to moisture vapour; impervious to liquids and bacteria; promote angiogenesis; promote granulation; protect the wound
Alginates	Provide a moist wound healing environment; absorb significant amounts of exudate; easily removed by irrigation techniques; comfortable; haemostatic properties are reported (but not in every alginate)
Low adherent	Generally used as a secondary dressing; it may, however, be used as a primary dressing
Hydrofibre	Moist wound environment; management of a large amount of exudate; non-adherent

Adapted from Collier, 1996

Key points

❖ A complex set of events occurs upon injury to the skin, which appear to be relatively simple but, in fact, are exceptionally complicated giving rise to physical and chemical reactions and cellular episodes.

❖ The ideal wound temperature has been identified as 37°C.

❖ A huge array of dressing products are currently on the market which can be confusing to the nurse trying to decide which product to use.

References

Adzick NS, Harrison MR, Glick PL (1985) Comparison of fetal and adult wound healing by histological, enzyme-histochemical and hydroxide proline determinations. *J Pediatr Surg* **20**(4): 315–19

Bond S (1998) Eating matter — improving dietary care in hospitals. *Nurs Standard* **12**(17): 41–2

Brunner L, Suddarth D (1992) *Textbook of Adult Nursing*. Chapman and Hall, London

Butterworth RJ, Jansi B, Hughes LE (1992) *Persistent inflammation — good healing*. Proceedings of the 2nd European Conference on Advances in Wound Management, Macmillan Magazines, London: 11–12

Chen J, Hutchinson J (1998) *Aquacel Hydrofibre Dressing: The Next Step in Wound Dressing Technology*. Churchill Communications, Europe, London

Chen WYJ, Rogers AA (1992) Characterization of biologic properties of wound fluid collected during early stages of wound healing. *J Invest Dermatol* **99**: 559–64

Collier M (1996) The principles of optimum wound management. *Nurs Standard* **10**(43): 47–52

Davis M, Dunkley P, Harden RM, Harding K, Laidlaw JM, Morris A, Wood RAB (1992) *The Wound Management Programme Centre for Medical Education*. Ninewells Hospital and Medical School, University of Dundee

Dealey C (1994) *The Care of Wounds*. Blackwell Scientific, London: 65–82

Eaglstein WH 1985) The effect of occlusive dressings on collagen synthesis and re-epithelialisation in superficial wounds. In: Ryan TJ, ed *An Environment for Healing: The Role of Occlusion*. International Congress and Symposium Series No 88. Royal Society of Medicine, London: 31–8

Ferguson M (1993) Wound healing and ageing. In: Bennett G, Moody M, eds. *Wound Care for Health Professionals*. Chapman and Hall, London: 13–33

Field C, Kerstein M (1994) Overview of wound healing in a moist environment. *Am J Surg* **167**(suppl 1a): 25–65

Flanagan M (1996) A practical framework for wound assessment 1: physiology. *Br J Nurs* **5**(22): 1391–7

Flanagan M (1997a) *Wound Healing*. Churchill Livingstone, Edinburgh

Flanagan M (1997b) Wound healing and management. *Primary Health Care* **7**(4): 31–9

Gilge O (1948) Ulcus cruris in venous circulatory disturbances. *Acta Dermato-Venered* **29**(Suppl 22): 13–28

Grinnell F, Zhu MF (1994) Identification of neurtrophil elastase as the proteinase in burn wound fluid responsible for degradation of fibonectin. *J Invest Dermatol* **103**: 155–91

Grinnell F, Zhu MF (1996) Fribronectin degradagion in chronic wounds depends on the relative levels of elastase and 1-proteinase inhibitor, and 2-macroglobulin. *J Invest Dermatol* **106**: 335–41

Heffernan A, Martin AJ (1994) A comparison of a modified form of Granuflex and a conventional dressing in the management of lacerations, abrasions and minor operations wounds in an accident and emergency department. *J Accid Emerg Med* **11**: 227–30

Hopkinson I (1992) Growth factors and extracellular matrix. *J Wound Care* **1**(2): 47–50

Irvin TT, Challopadhyay DK (1978) Asorbic acid requirements in post-operative patients. *Am J Surg* **47**: 49

Kerstein MD (1997) The scientific basis of healing. *Adv Wound Management* **10**(3): 30–6

Knighton D, Hunt T, Scheunstuhl H (1983) Oxygen tension regulates the expression of angiogenesis factor by macrophages. *Science* **221**: 1283–5

Lamke LO, Nilsson CE (1997) The evaporative water loss from burns and water vapour permeability of grafts and artificial membranes used in treatment of burns. *Burns* **3**: 159–65

Lock PM (1980) The effects of temperature on mitotic activity at the edge of experimental wounds. In: Lundgren A, Soner AB, eds. *Symposia on Wound Healing: Plastic Surgical and Dermatologic Aspects*. Molndal, Sweden

Lydon M, Hutchinson J (1989) Dissolution of wound coagulum and promotion of granulation tissue under Duoderm. *Wounds* **1**: 95–106

McCaffrey M (1983) *Nursing the Patient in Pain*. Harper and Row, London

Madden MR, Finkelstein JL (1989) Comparison of an occlusive and semi-occlusive dressing and the effect of wound exudate upon keratincytes proliferation. *J Trauma* **29**: 924–30

Miller M, Collier M (1996) Understanding wounds. *Professional Nurse* (supplement). In association with Johnson & Johnson Medical, EMAP Healthcare, London

Morsion MJ (1992) *A Colour Guide to Nursing Management of Wounds*. Wolfe, London: 1–47

Morison M, Moffat C, Bridel-Nixon J, Bale S (1997) *Nursing Management of Chronic Wounds*. 2nd edn. Mosby, London: 1–26

Newmeth AJ, Eaglstein WH (1991) Faster healing and less pain in skin biopsy sites treated with an occlusive dressing. *Arch Dermatol* **127**: 1679–83

Ono I, Gunji H (1994) Evaluation of cytokines in donor site wound fluids. *Scand J Plast Reconstr Surg Hand Surg* **28**: 269–73

Roberts A, McLoughlin B (1997) Abstract 7th European Conference on Advances in Wound Management. In: Leapter D, Dealey C, Franks P, Hofman D, Moffatt CJ, eds. EMAP Healthcare Conferences, London: 150

Roberts C (1998) Wound management products — the evidence we need and the difficulties in obtaining it. *J Tissue Viabil* **8**(2): 12–15

Rogers AA, Burnett S, Moore JC, Shakespeare PG, Chen WYJ (1995) Involvement of proteolytic enzymes, plasminogen activators and matrix metalloproteinases in the pathophysiology of pressure ulcers. *Wound Repair Regeneration* **3**: 273–83

Siegal DM (1996) Surgical paeval: a novel cost-effective approach to wound closure and dressings. *J Am Acad Dermatol* **34**: 673–5

Silver IA (1992) Advances in the physiology of wound healing. 2nd European Conference on Advances in Wound Management. Macmillan Magazines, London: 1–4

Silver IA (1994) The physiology of wound healing. *J Wound Care* **3**(2): 106–9

Thomas S (1990) *Wound Management and Dressings*. Pharmaceutical Press, London

Thomas S (1997) Wound management and dressings. Assessment and management of wound exudate. *J Wound Care* **6**(7): 327–30

Tortora G, Anagnostakos NP (1987) *Anatomy and Physiology Biological Sciences*. 5th edn. Harper and Row, International Edition, New York: 101–4

Waugh L (1990) *Psychological Aspects of Cancer Pain. Staff Nurses' Survival Guide*. The Professional Series, Austen Cornish, London: 194–201

Winter GD (1962) Formulation of the scab and the rate of epithelialization in the skin of the domestic pig. *Nature* **193**: 293–4

Winter GD (1975) Epidermal wound healing. In: Turner TD, Brain KR, eds. *Surgical Dressings in Hospital Environment*. Proceedings of Conference, Cardiff, Surgical Dressings Research Unit, Welsh School of Pharmacy

Wysocki AB (1996) Wound fluids and the pathogenesis of chronic wounds. *J Wound Ostomy Continence Nurse* **23**: 283–90

2

A topical issue: the use of antibacterials in wound pathogen control

Richard White, Rose Cooper, Andrew Kingsley

Introduction

Intact skin provides a physical barrier to the ingress of micro-organisms, but once it is breached by wounding, micro-organisms from the surrounding skin, other body sites, or from exogenous sources have access to the internal warm and moist environment. Whether organisms then survive depends on their ability to evade the body's immune response, and whether their essential chemical and physical requirements for survival are met. Transient wound contaminants may not persist, but those species that do grow and divide may establish a spectrum of conditions between wound colonisation and wound infection (Kingsley, 2001a). A multitude of complex influences, such as the size, position and duration of a wound, local dissolved oxygen levels and host immuno-competency are balanced against number and type of invading microbial species and the presence of foreign bodies (including necrotic tissue and eschar) in determining the outcome (Emmerson, 1998). Numbers and types of micro-organisms in wounds are never uniform (Cooper and Lawrence, 1996a), and acute wounds may contain communities distinct from those in chronic wounds (Bowler and Davies, 1999). Microbial inhabitants of wounds have long been identified and enumerated, but neither the extent of their interactions within the wound environment nor their influences on the healing process have yet been fully characterised. This chapter attempts to evaluate the current evidence on the importance of managing wound bioburden, with a view to the early recognition of patients at risk of infection, and the selection of appropriate topical antimicrobial intervention to prevent delayed healing.

Wound microbiology

Investigations into the microbial flora of wounds began in 1874 when Billroth detected streptococci in wounds. Koch noticed staphylococci in pus in 1878 and Pasteur cultivated them in 1880, but it was Alexander Ogston, in 1881, who realised that they were associated with acute and chronic abscesses. Since the nineteenth century improvements in techniques have allowed the recovery, identification and enumeration of a wide variety of microbial species from wounds. It is clear that many wounds support relatively stable, mixed communities of micro-organisms, often without signs of clinical infection (Hansson and Faergemann, 1995), yet despite extensive investigations into the effects of micro-organisms in wounds, a consensus of their impact on the wound healing process is not yet agreed (Bowler *et al*, 2001).

The importance of microbial numbers in wound infection

French military surgeons during World War I recognised that wounds containing high numbers of micro-organisms (or low numbers of streptococci) were prone to infection and should be healed by secondary intention (Hepburn, 1919). Elek (1956) showed that introducing 7.5×10^6 staphylococci into normal skin induced pustule formation and that similar effects were caused by lower bacterial numbers when skin was compromised by sutures. Teplitz *et al* (1964) studied the effect of *Pseudomonas aeruginosa* in burns created in rats, and found that 10^5 cfu/g induced invasion and systemic sepsis. Although definitions of wound infection vary (Leaper, 1999), there is sufficient evidence to demonstrate a relationship between elevated microbial numbers and wound infection (Bornside and Bornside, 1979; Lookingbill *et al*, 1978; Raahave *et al*, 1986; Breidenbach and Trager, 1995). Furthermore, failure of skin grafts in wounds with elevated bacterial populations (Teplitz *et al*, 1964; Krizek *et al*, 1967; Robson and Heggers, 1969; Robson and Heggers, 1970) has also contributed to the general acceptance that a wound bioburden of 10^5 cfu/g or cm^2 indicates an infected wound (or 10^4 cfu/g in complex extremity wounds, Breidenbach and Trager, 1995), and that population sizes below this level are required for successful grafting.

The impact of infection on wound healing

Although studies have indicated that infected wounds exhibited accelerated healing (Tenorio *et al*, 1976; Raju *et al*, 1977), most studies have shown the reverse. The development of clinical infection usually interrupts the normal healing process (Bucknall, 1980; de Haan *et al*, 1974; Robson *et al*, 1990) and repeated trauma, ischaemia and infection are leading causes of wound chronicity (Tarnuzzer and Schultz, 1996). Repeated infection causes elevated levels of pro-inflammatory cytokines and metalloproteinases, while bacterial enzymes degrade growth factors and extracellular matrix components, and cytotoxic bacterial toxins impair the function of many human cells intimately involved in the wound repair process. The relationship between microbial population size and delayed wound healing was first investigated in pressure sores, where reduction to levels below 10^6 cfu/ml of wound exudate was required for wound healing to progress (Bendy *et al*, 1964). Another undesirable effect attributed to the presence of micro-organisms in wounds is that anaerobic bacteria can give rise to malodorous wounds (Bowler *et al*, 1999b).

Until the advent of Lister's antiseptic surgery, Galen's concept of laudable pus was generally accepted, and the development of wound infection was encouraged. Now the deleterious effects of wound infection in interrupting healing are more clearly understood and so there are compelling reasons to reduce the microbial load in wounds when skin grafts are required, or where infection and/or malodours develop.

The impact of specific microbial species on healing

The involvement of specific micro-organisms in delayed healing has also been extensively studied. *Staphylococcus aureus* is the organism most frequently isolated from wounds, yet there are conflicting reports of its clinical significance. Undoubtedly it has the potential to cause infections, but it can also colonise wounds. Daltrey *et al* (1981) showed that *Staphylococcus aureus* was not associated with any trend in delayed healing, and in reviewing previous studies Bowler (1998) deduced that there was no correlation between the presence of this organism and wound infection. Madson *et al* (1996) reported that both beta haemolytic streptococci and *Staphylococcus aureus* did contribute to delayed healing. The destructive effect of beta haemolytic streptococci to skin grafts was recognised by plastic surgeons in the 1950s (Jackson *et al*, 1951), and the need to utilise antimicrobial therapy to ensure their removal from chronic leg ulcers before grafting was recently reinforced (Schraibman, 1990). *Pseudomonas aeruginosa* has been linked to enlarged venous ulcers with delayed healing (Madsen *et al*, 1996) and to enlarging pressure sores (Daltrey *et al*, 1981). This opportunist pathogen possesses a variety of virulence determinants (Lyczak *et al*, 2000), whose expression is influenced by population density. Another group of bacteria that have the potential to impinge on healing is the anaerobic bacteria; these possess significant virulence factors (Duerdin, 1994), and there is a correlation between the incidence of anaerobes and chronic wound infection (Bowler and Davies, 1999b; Bowler *et al*, 2001). Despite all of these observations, Trengove *et al* (1996) was unable to associate any particular type of bacterium with delayed healing, although the presence of four or more groups of bacteria did retard healing. It is possible that synergistic relationships between different species might enhance their effects on wound healing, and so there are valid arguments to reduce the levels of specific organisms in wounds, as well as total bioburden.

The impact of colonisation on wound healing

Whether healing in colonised wounds is influenced by bioburden is not clear. Halbert *et al* (1992) concluded that venous ulcers colonised by bacteria were of longer duration than those without, but it has been suggested that the microbial flora in wounds without signs of clinical infection does not influence healing

(Hansson *et al*, 1995). The concept that, 'as a rule the bacteria in ulcers are saprophytic and will disappear when the favourable environment for their growth is lost' (Eriksson *et al*, 1984) demonstrates that not all microbial loads in wounds are harmful, and it is imperative that antimicrobial agents be used discriminatorily.

Antimicrobial control strategies

The use of chemicals to control the growth of micro-organisms in wounds has a long history, and a wide range of agents is available. Antibiotics exploit structural and functional differences between host and microbial cells, and exert relatively high selective toxicity by targeting a specific microbial process. Both antiseptics and disinfectants possess a broad spectrum of activity by non-specifically affecting multiple intracellular target sites, and therefore exhibit lower selective toxicity. Microbial inhibition is achieved by either inducing lethal events (cidal agents) or by interrupting growth without loss of viability (static agents). The removal or inactivation of static agents curtails their inhibitory effect and allows microbial growth to resume. As well as contact time, concentration and the presence of organic matter may influence the effectiveness of an anti-microbial agent, and these factors need consideration in wound management. Systemic antibiotic regimes are designed to maintain appropriate tissue and serum concentrations, but levels of topical agents will fluctuate between applications, unless sustained release systems are employed.

The literature appears to contain some mixed messages about the use of antibiotics, which can probably be attributed to varying interpretation of the terms colonised, infected or clinically infected and routine. There is limited evidence, for example, that the routine use of systemic antibiotics in the management of clinically infected leg ulcers is of no benefit (Alinovi *et al*, 1986). Whereas appropriately selected antibiotics are valuable in the treatment of wounds with spreading infection (Bowler *et al*, 2001), the **routine** use of systemic antibiotics for chronic wounds without clinical infection is not recommended (O'Meara *et al*, 2001). Furthermore, the use of **topical** antibiotics is not justified for the routine treatment of colonised or infected wounds (Drug and Therapeutics Bulletin, 1991). Topical antibiotics can provoke delayed hyper-sensitivity reactions (Zaki *et al*, 1994), allow colonisation by resistant organisms (Huovinen *et al*, 1994), and select for resistance (*British Medical Journal*, 1977). This is particularly evident with those antibiotics that are used both topically and systemically, eg. gentamicin, metronidazole, sodium fusidate, chlortetracycline and others. Resistance to antibiotics has become a serious problem for those involved in wound care; the situation has been described as 'crisis' in the USA (Colsky *et al*, 1998). Both colonised and infected wounds act as a reservoir of potential pathogens that may contribute to increased risks of cross-infection, and the presence of resistant strains is an additional problem. Appropriate management of these problems by healthcare professionals is crucial.

Active steps taken to reduce colonisation or counter infection depend upon the nature of the wound, status of the patient, and the pathogenicity of the organism(s) involved. Clearly, an organ transplant patient threatened with a methicillin-resistant *Staphylococcus aureus* (MRSA) infection in their surgical wound is at greater risk, as their immunosuppressed status puts them at high risk of life-threatening infection, than one with a long-standing leg ulcer known to be colonised but with minimal host reaction. Antimicrobial intervention in such vulnerable patients should always be sooner than in immunocompetent individuals.

Whereas some topical antimicrobials may be beneficial (O'Meara *et al*, 2001), the effects of antiseptics are variable. Fifteen-minute exposure of venous leg ulcers to dressings impregnated with four different antiseptics has been shown to reduce mean numbers of bacteria per ulcer, but not all bacteria gave statistically significant reductions (Hansson and Faergemann, 1995).

As elective wounds are usually subject to rigorous pre-operative antiseptic measures and aseptic surgical techniques, infection is minimised and healing often proceeds within the expected time-frame. Traumatic wounds are more likely to contain devitalised tissue and debris, and to be contaminated with micro-organisms from environmental sources. Consequently, infection rates are higher. Chronic wounds such as leg ulcers (Dale *et al*, 1983) or pressure sores (Daltrey *et al*, 1981) are inevitably colonised with a mixture of species and many of these are potential pathogens; progression to infection in chronic wounds usually reflects host susceptibility.

The benefits of reducing microbial loads in wounds include the prevention of clinical infection with concomitant delays in healing, the removal of organisms destructive to skin grafts, and the removal of organisms that generate malodours. Even the mechanical reduction in bioburden effected by wound rinsing is significant, but without antimicrobial agents population densities are quickly recovered.

Definitions

Definitions of commonly used terms in the field of infection control are provided to avoid ambiguity (*Table 2.1*).

The accepted diagnostic criteria for wound infection are:

- abscess
- cellulitis
- discharge
- delayed healing
- discolouration
- friable, bleeding granulation tissue
- unexpected pain/tenderness
- pocketing/bridging at base of the wound
- abnormal smell
- wound breakdown.

An infected wound may not have all of these signs (Cutting and Harding, 1994), but in the majority of cases cellulitis will be present indicating invasion of the tissues surrounding the wound bed. The continuum of infection is illustrated in *Figure 2.2*.

Table 2.1: Definitions of terms
Antibiotic: A chemical derived from a micro-organism which has the capacity, in dilute solutions, to selectively inhibit the growth (static) of, or to kill (cidal) other micro-organisms
Disinfectant: A non-selective agent (sometimes combined with detergent) that destroys, removes or inactivates potential pathogens on inert surfaces. It is used particularly on instruments, work surfaces and patient contact equipment but not intended for use on the tissues of the body where toxicity would impair healing. Different disinfectants will have differing activity against different microbial species, and so should be appropriately selected for the expected contaminating pathogens
Antiseptic: An antiseptic can be a diluted disinfectant; it is a substance that can be used on skin and on wounds to either kill or prevent the multiplication of potentially pathogenic organisms. Antiseptics have the advantage of rarely selecting for resistant microbial strains, and, being topical, do not rely on the bloodstream for access to the wound. This is particularly important in ischaemic wounds (Saffle and Schnebly, 1994). However they have the disadvantage of low selectivity and may possess toxicity to host tissues at higher concentrations (Scott Ward and Saffle, 1995)
Bioburden: The microbial loading of the skin and/or wounds with normal commensals and potential pathogens
Colonisation: The presence of multiplying bacteria with no overt host (immunological) reaction (Ayton, 1985) or clinical symptoms. This definition currently applies irrespective of the numbers and species or organisms present in the wound
Critical colonisation: A term applied to the situation where host defences fail to maintain the balance of organisms in a wound at colonisation (Kingsley, 2001a). Typically the wound is indolent and expresses some of the clinical symptoms characteristic of infection, such as increased exudate and surface slough or odour, without visible cellulitis in the surrounding skin, sudden necrosis or extension in the wound itself
Infection: The presence of multiplying bacteria in body tissues, resulting in spreading cellular injury due to competitive metabolism, toxins, intracellular replication or antigen-antibody response (host reaction). This would be apparent as any one or more of the classical signs of inflammation, ie. erythema, heat, swelling, pain

Measures designed to prevent wound infection

Measures to prevent wound infection and delayed healing situations are based on sound tissue viability principles. These are:

- Identify aetiology of wound.
- Remove any continuing intrinsic and extrinsic causative factors such as venous hypertension and shearing pressure.

⌘ Eliminate or reduce any factors that may impair healing such as malnutrition, hyperglycaemia, anaemia amongst others.

⌘ Initiate most effective therapy at outset; do not use holding or 'wait and see' treatments because they are more convenient.

⌘ Utilise universal infection control precautions to prevent cross contamination from the wound.

⌘ Remove necrotic and foreign material.

⌘ Allow drainage of wound exudate/pus in particular from sinuses (this does not preclude use of occlusive dressings but does help to determine dressing frequency dependent on the absorbency of the individual product.

⌘ Observe closely for signs of change at all dressing changes; in particular those representing a delay in healing or infection.

⌘ Construct a care plan that details expected progress so that delays can be detected at the earliest opportunity.

⌘ Use a framework to guide decision making for undesired events (Kingsley, 2001a).

Modern 'moist wound healing' dressings have been shown to be valuable in infection control. They form part of the non-microbiological approach to control the wound bioburden. Some occlusive dressings such as hydrocolloids have both bacterial and viral barrier properties; these can be used to 'contain' pathogens within the wound environment so reducing the probability of spread and cross-infection (Bowler *et al*, 1993). Hydrocolloids have also been shown to reduce the airborne distribution of organisms, through aerosol formation, at dressing change (Lawrence, 1994). In general, occlusive dressings are associated with a lower overall wound infection rate than non-occlusive dressings (Hutchinson and Lawrence, 1991). Dry dressings such as gauzes stick to the wound and may leave contaminating fibres that act as foci for infection. On removal, their traumatic detachment has been demonstrated to spread bacteria by aerosol formation (Lawrence *et al*, 1992). In hospital clinics this is likely to be a factor in the spread of infections. Whilst there is no evidence that traditional, dry dressings have any role in infection control and may even lead to an increased rate of infection, some modern dressings have evidence to support their use in this context. A novel hydrofibre dressing, Aquacel (ConvaTec), has been found to bind bacteria and thereby 'contain' the spread of pathogens. In a study using an *in vitro* wound model seeded with *Staphylococcus aureus*, Bowler *et al* (1999a) have compared a number of similar fibrous dressings. Results show Aquacel to be most effective in binding bacteria (p<0.001), followed by alginates Algosteril (Beiersdorf) and Kaltostat (ConvaTec).

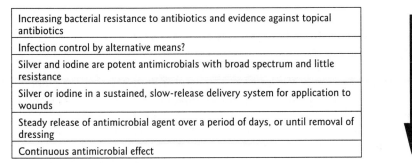

| Increasing bacterial resistance to antibiotics and evidence against topical antibiotics |
| Infection control by alternative means? |
| Silver and iodine are potent antimicrobials with broad spectrum and little resistance |
| Silver or iodine in a sustained, slow-release delivery system for application to wounds |
| Steady release of antimicrobial agent over a period of days, or until removal of dressing |
| Continuous antimicrobial effect |

Figure 2.1: The role of silver- and iodine-impregnated dressings in topical antisepsis of critically colonised and infected wounds. The arrow indicates the thought/decision-making pathway

Type of wound	Acute	Acute	Acute and chronic	Acute and chronic	Acute and chronic
Wound status	Sterile	Contamination	Colonisation	Critical colonisation	Infection
Wound bioburden	Absent	Usually low numbers with little active growth (high in some trauma wounds)	A relatively stable, dynamic equilibrium	Host defences unable to maintain colonisation	Increased levels of pathogens and invasion into host tissues
Microbial diversity (ie. variety of species)	Absent	Restricted, mostly transient species	Wide range of commensals and potential pathogens	Similar to colonisation	Restricted
Indicators of clinical infection	Absent	Absent, except inflammation associated with trauma	No overt host response	Some indicators present	Present
Antimicrobial intervention strategies	None	Wound cleansing and removal of devitalised tissue and inanimate objects from trauma wounds. Prevent further contamination in burns	Usually none, except reduce β haem. Strep and pseudomonads prior to grafting. Topical agents for odour control	Topical antimicrobial agents	Systemic antibodies +/- topical anti-microbial agents

Figure 2.2: The infection continuum (adapted from Kingsley, 2001a)

Clinical evidence for the use of topical antiseptics

For many, the use of antiseptics in wound care is biased by the 'bad press' given to EUSOL (Edinburgh University Solution of Lime) and the confusion over iodine compounds. The value and use of EUSOL has led to vigorous debate and polarisation of healthcare professionals into a majority that vehemently oppose its use under any circumstances (Leaper, 1992) and a minority that still regard it as useful. The value and use of topical antiseptics in wound care has been debated for many years. In the UK in particular, the use of hypochlorites such as EUSOL is controversial (Moore, 1992). The consensus on EUSOL, especially amongst nurses, is that it has no place in wound care, regardless of the concentration used (Roe *et al*, 1994). This view is based on evidence that it is rapidly de-activated in the presence of pus, is painful to the patient, and delays healing by damaging cells and capillaries (Leaper, 1988). Iodine compounds have also attracted criticism (Rodeheaver, 1988). The main argument against the use of such agents is their potential toxicity (Lawrence, 1998a) — a factor related to concentration and exposure — and the attendant delay in healing compared to untreated controls (Brennan and Leaper, 1985).

Careful and objective review of the literature reveals that the use of many antiseptics in wound management must be subject to a risk-benefit assessment of possible local toxicity with beneficial antibacterial action (Kaye, 2000). Brennan and Leaper (1985) advise balancing the beneficial antimicrobial effects and bioavailability with possible cellular toxicity before usage.

In solution form, antiseptics are used to irrigate or cleanse the wound. This, by definition, means a short period of contact with the tissues. Solutions are, therefore, concentrated in order to have the desired effect — which increases the likelihood of tissue toxicity and delayed healing. Antiseptic agents incorporated into dressings are in contact for much longer, and can be more dilute, less toxic and exert a prolonged antimicrobial effect.

The ideal antiseptic will have the following key attributes (adapted from Morison, 1990):

- broad spectrum of activity
- low potential for resistance
- non-toxic: to white blood cells in the early inflammatory stage and later to fibroblasts and keratinocytes
- rapid acting
- neither irritant nor a sensitiser
- effective, even in the presence of exudate, pus, slough etc.

Iodine

Iodine, particularly in the safe, modern iodophor povidone-iodine (a polyvinyl pyrrolidone surfactant/iodine complex or PVP-I) and cadexomer (a three-dimensional starch lattice containing iodine) is a very useful bacteriostatic and bactericidal agent being active against MRSA and other pathogens (Mertz *et al*, 1999). The use of PVP-I as a pre-surgical skin antiseptic is unquestioned although its value in wound antisepsis is subject to debate (Thomas, 1988; Rodeheaver, 1988; Goldenheim, 1993; Lawrence, 1998a/b; Gulliver, 1999). Concerns about toxicity and impaired healing relate mainly to the older products that contain elemental iodine, although PVP-I is also implicated (Kramer, 1999). The newer products, eg. Ioban (3M), Inadine (J&J Medical), Iodosorb (Smith & Nephew), appear to be safer and have a very wide spectrum of activity (Gilchrist 1997a; Sundberg and Meller, 1997). In the USA, the Food and Drug

Administration maintains that PVP-I in 5–10% solutions do not adversely affect healing (Federal Register, 1994) although a later review of published data by Kramer (1999) disputes this.

Iodine iodophor is available in a range of concentrations as medicated dressings (eg. Inadine, Iodoflex, Smith & Nephew), solutions and ointments (eg. Betadine, SSL), powder and spray (eg. Savlon Dry powder, Novartis), and incise drapes (Ioban). PVP-I gradually releases free iodine that has a broad spectrum of antimicrobial activity, including MRSA (McLure and Gordon, 1992; Lawrence, 1998b). The slow release from the iodophor is intended to optimise activity and to reduce toxicity.

The cadexomer is a polysaccharide starch lattice containing 0.9% elemental iodine that is released on exposure to exudate (Lawrence, 1998a) and has antimicrobial activity for up to three days (Mertz *et al*, 1999). It has been extensively evaluated in a variety of acute and chronic wounds and found to be safe and effective (Sundberg and Meller, 1997). The PVP-I containing dressings such as Inadine (a sterile knitted viscose dressing impregnated with 10% PVP-I in a water-soluble base) and Ioban (iodophor incorporated onto a film) provide sustained release of low levels of free iodine. This and other modern iodinated dressings should only be used on exuding wounds for best effect.

Iodine is also available as the alcoholic tincture and as iodoform, neither is regarded as being valuable in wound management because of pain and limited antibacterial activity respectively.

Silver

Silver and silver compounds have been routinely used as bactericidals for over a century. It is generally recognised as a safe, broad spectrum agent with only irritation and skin discolouration (argyria) reported for the inorganic nitrate solution (Wright *et al*, 1998a). Silver acts as a heavy metal by impairing the bacterial electron transport system and some DNA functions (Russell and Hugo, 1994; Cervantes and Silver, 1996). To do this, the 'active' agents, silver ions, have to be bioavailable (ie. to be able to enter the cell), at the correct concentration in solution (Demling and DeSanti, 2001).

Silver nitrate was probably the first silver compound used on wounds where it has an astringent and irritating effect; because of these problems and lack of evidence it is rarely used today except for the occasional use in reducing hypergranulation. The esterification (chemical bonding) of silver with a sulphonamide antimicrobial, sulphadiazine, (silver sulphadiazine or SSD) has resulted in a very safe, broad-spectrum agent for topical use. Silver is released slowly from the oil-in-water cream formulation in concentrations that are selectively toxic to micro-organisms such as bacteria (MRSA, gentamicin-resistant pseudomonads and enterococci) and fungi (Goodman and Gilman, 1990).

Best known as the Flamazine 1% cream, SSD has been a mainstay of topical burns therapy (Pruitt, 1987) and has been used successfully in acute (Buckley *et al*, 2000) and chronic wounds (Bishop *et al*, 1992) to treat infection. Resistance to SSD has been reported (Modak and Fox, 1981) but is rare. A variety of topical silver preparations have been evaluated on chronic wounds (O'Meara *et al*, 2000, and 2001) in controlled trials with generally favourable results.

Recently a number of silver-containing dressings have become available (Adams *et al*, 1999; Furr *et al*, 1994; Williams, 1994; Williams, 1997; Wright *et al*, 1998a/b; Yin *et al*, 1999). In any formulation, the way in which silver is incorporated and how it interacts with micro-organisms, ie. its bioavailability in solution is critical in determining its antimicrobial efficiency and its safety (Demling and DeSanti, 2001). Actisorb Plus (recently renamed Actisorb Silver 220, J&J Medical) contains silver impregnated onto an activated charcoal cloth (Williams, 1994). It is claimed to be effective against a wide range of micro-organisms (Furr *et al*, 1994). There are numerous reports of clinical data to support the clinical efficacy of Actisorb Silver 220 (Bornier and Jeannin, 1989; Millward, 1991; Wunderlich and Orfanos, 1991; Tebbe and Orfanos, 1994; Cassino *et al*, 2001; Scanlon and Dowsett, 2001; White, 2001). Arglaes (Maersk Medical) is available as a slow-release film dressing polymer with silver ions (Williams, 1997). Acticoat film (Westaim Co, now available from Smith & Nephew in the UK) is an antimicrobial barrier dressing which has also been shown to be effective against a wide range of organisms (Yin *et al*, 1999).

Although the delivery systems vary, the mode of action principle is the same in each case. There is currently very little clinical evidence available to support these products; their rationale is based on *in vitro* studies (Furr *et al*, 1994; Wright *et al*, 1998b). Preliminary findings from an *in vitro* wound model (Bowler *et al*, 2000) suggests that not all can be expected to be equally effective. In heavily exuding wounds, the proteinaceous material in wound fluid may bind to the charcoal layer in Actisorb Silver 220 so reducing the release of silver and thereby the antibacterial activity. These *in vitro* findings question the capacity of this dressing to inhibit wound bacteria in clinical practice (Bowler *et al*, 2000), although clinical data suggests otherwise. Evaluation of the antimicrobial activity of such 'medicated' dressings *in vivo* on colonised or infected wounds is technically difficult. Products that can sustain the interaction of silver with micro-organisms in the exuding wound are likely to be more effective in controlling infection. *Figure 2.1* illustrates the rationale for iodine and silver dressings in the treatment of critically colonised and infected wounds.

Honey

The use of honey in wound care is largely confined to wounds healing by secondary intent. Historically, honeys have been used in this context for thousands of years (Jones, 2001), and recently there has been a resurgence of interest in honey. This was prompted mainly by the laboratory demonstration of its antimicrobial efficacy on wound pathogens (Willix *et al*, 1992; Cooper and Molan, 1999; Cooper *et al*, 1999), and its clinical effect on selected patients (Dunford *et al*, 2000; Natarajan *et al*, 2001; Cooper *et al*, 2001). Antibacterial properties of honey and its potential in the treatment of wounds has been extensively reviewed by Molan (1992 and 1999 respectively). The mechanisms by which honey influences the wound healing process are currently incompletely elucidated (Tonks *et al*, 2001), and until further clinical evidence is accumulated, honey is unlikely to be widely accepted by healthcare professionals.

Proflavine

Proflavine is an acridine derivative (a compound originally used in the manufacture of dyes) available as a cream British Pharmaceutical Codex (BPC), solution BPC and as the hemisulphate. This has been in use for many years as a slow acting, mildly bacteriostatic (ie. inhibits bacterial growth) agent in wound management. In particular, proflavine is still widely used prophylactically as a gauze soak for wound packing even though it has been found to be inferior to an alginate dressing in this respect (Gupta *et al*, 1991). There is no reliable evidence that it is effective in this respect, or that it has any clinical benefits. Indeed, there are reports of mutagenicity (gene and chromosomal mutations) of proflavine on bacterial (Iwamoto *et al*, 1992) and cell cultures (DeMarini *et al*, 1988), raising profound questions about its safety.

Chlorhexidine compounds

These are useful antiseptics for skin being highly effective for hand washing and surgical scrub. They bind to the stratum corneum and have a persisting activity, remaining active for at least six hours after application (Kaye, 2000). The acetate, Chlorasept (Baxter), is intended for wound irrigation. The gluconate is active against gram-negative organisms such as *Pseudomonas aeruginosa* and gram-positives such as *Staphylococcus aureus* and *Escherichia coli*. Their toxicity and use on wounds has not been established categorically, although they may be a useful therapeutic option as an agent for topical use (Scott Ward and Saffle, 1995).

Hydrogen peroxide

Usually used as a 3% (10 volumes) or 6% (20 volumes) aqueous solution to clean necrotic, infected wounds and those contaminated with soil and foreign particles, hydrogen peroxide is antiseptic due to the release of oxygen, an oxidising agent, on contact with the tissues. There are safety concerns about using hydrogen peroxide solutions on open wounds because of reports of tissue embolism (Scott Ward and Saffle, 1995). Hydrogen peroxide is also available as a 1.5% cream (Hioxyl, Quinoderm) for desloughing wounds but without clinical evidence to support or refute its efficacy.

Potassium permanganate

Weak solutions of this oxidising agent (1 part in 5000 — 1 in 10,000) are used as soaks to cleanse and deodorise eczematous wounds and leg ulcers. Although favoured by dermatologists, there is no evidence published to support their use (Roe and Cullum, 1995).

Wound cleansing

The value of cleansing wounds rests with the removal of excess exudate, foreign bodies including dressing residues, necrotic tissue, loose slough and wound edge crusting (which is fibrin, dehydrated exudate and dressing residue). Removal of all these and leaving the wound moist will ensure that healing will be assisted to progress unhindered. Cleaning that does not seek to achieve any of these aims is unlikely to be of value and is more likely to cause harm by damaging fragile new tissue growth, thereby delaying healing. However, if one considers wound cleaning to include the peri-wound skin then removal of exudate and dressing adhesive residues should reduce the likelihood of maceration, which can extend wounds (Cutting, 1999), and excoriation from exudate enzymes, bacterial toxins and skin pH disturbance.

The ideal method of cleansing depends on the individual circumstances of the case. Some may require rapid sharp debridement under anaesthetic whilst in others this may not be suitable and more conservative approaches are needed. Though debridement is technically cleansing, it is usually considered separately. Normally cleansing is achieved by irrigation with a fluid, or mechanically with a moistened wipe. For wounds healing by secondary intention the fluid can be sterile normal saline as it is isotonic but this is expensive in comparison to tap water which is the fluid of first choice. Studies on traumatic wounds by Hall Angeras *et al* (1992) suggest that there is no quantifiable infection risk with tap water. The use of tap water makes cleansing convenient as it can be done in a sink under running water, in the bath or shower or, for leg ulcers, in a bucket. These processes have the added advantage of ease of cleaning surrounding skin. Pressurised irrigation can be achieved notably with commercially available aerosol spray cans. The pressure must be adequate to dislodge loose debris and slough without causing tissue damage. Whirlpool baths, for example, may cause damage to tissues in leg wounds (Oliver, 1997), and increase the risks of pseudomonal follicullitis. Spray cans deliver a pressurised stream of saline at 8 pounds per square inch (55kPa), which is considered optimum for effectiveness. Such a delivery by aerosols onto the flat surface of most wounds offers a high risk for cross contamination of both the practitioner and surrounding environment, making them inadvisable for use anywhere but the home (avoids nosocomial infection risk) with suitable protective clothing. To improve these devices a disposable splash guard would make them more viable. Microbial colonisation of open wounds is inevitable and cleansing can lower the bioburden transiently. The purpose of cleansing (whether pressurised or not and with whatever fluid) is to aid removal of necrotic tissues and foreign bodies which provide the medium for overgrowth, a phenomenon which can cause delay in healing. As for use of antiseptic solutions as enhanced cleansing agents, Thomlinson (1997) notes that the duration of contact is generally too short to be effective.

Wound dressings

Malodour is common in chronic wounds; it is associated with aerobic and anaerobic bacteria colonising or infecting the wound (Bowler *et al*, 1999b). The use of odour controlling dressings such as those containing charcoal (eg. Actisorb, Carboflex, Lyofoam C) can be very helpful (Thomas *et al*, 1998a). Only Carboflex, from this category, currently has the capacity to manage exudate (Thomas *et al*, 1998a) and still control odour effectively (Thomas *et al*, 1998b). This is attributable to an absorbent wound contact layer that manages the exudate, restricting exudate access to the charcoal adsorbent layer. Whilst odour control alone does not eradicate infection, or indeed, alter bacterial growth, it does have substantial patient quality of life benefits and should, therefore, be an adjunct to any topical and/or systemic antibacterial therapy (Haughton and Young, 1995). Honey may also have a role to play in the control of malodorous wounds (Dunford *et al*, 2000; Kingsley, 2001b).

The use of modern dressings in infection control shows great promise. Medicated (silver and iodine complexes) dressings can be useful in local control of bacterial bioburden provided the active agents (silver ions and elemental iodine) are available in solution at an appropriate concentration over time. Such dressings will, in turn, assist in infection control by reducing the numbers of wound pathogens available for cross-infection. Dressings containing antibiotics generally have a diminishing place in wound treatment due primarily to antibiotic resistance. However, a case can be made for the use of topical metronidazole gel in the palliative treatment of malodorous malignant (fungating) wounds where odour is a major problem, and because of the terminal nature of the disease, antibiotic resistance is not an issue (Rice, 1992).

Chronic wounds

The detailed reviews conducted by O'Meara *et al* (2000, 2001) and the Scottish Intercollegiate Guidelines Network (SIGN, 1998) have found little evidence to support the routine use of systemic antibiotics in patients with chronic wounds. Acute and spreading infections in chronic wounds should, however, be treated with systemic antibiotics (Bowler *et al*, 2001). Topical dressings, creams or ointments that provide a sufficient delivery of an antiseptic agent (eg. silver or iodine) may be useful (White *et al*, 2001). However, the use of povidone-iodine in solution as a wound cleanser is not justified (Leaper, 1994; Burks, 1998). Solutions used as rinses do not have sufficiently long contact time to be of much effect. Cleansers that rely on pressure, as in aerosol sprays of normal saline, or contain biocompatible surfactants to help remove necrotic material, are effective, but infection control measures should be carefully considered before use.

Surgical wounds

Clean surgery carries a small (1–5%) risk of post-operative wound infection whereas 'dirty procedures' such as that involving the large intestines has a much higher risk (up to 27%; Nichols, 1998). Minimising the incidence of infection relies on adequate asepsis, antisepsis and preservation of local host defences (Hunt, 1981). Asepsis involves effective infection control to minimise exogenous contamination during surgery. Antisepsis involves skin antiseptics and prophylactic antibiotics prior to surgery (Hansis, 1996). Recent guidelines on the prevention of surgical site infection have been published (Mangram, 1999). The emphasis on surgical wound healing is rapid perfusion as ischaemic tissue heals poorly and is easily infected (Hunt and Hopf, 1997). Healing and resistance to infection improve with increased local blood supply, and hence tissue oxygenation. Delivery of antibiotics, systemically dosed, to the infected wound also depends on perfusion. Antibiotics given at the time of injury will reduce, but not eliminate, the risk of infection. In one third of wound infections, bacteria cultured from the wound are susceptible to the prophylactic antibiotic provided; the key factors involved here are patients with hypoxia and local perfusion problems (Hunt and Hopf, 1997). In such instances, it is easy to make a case for prophylactic and therapeutic antiseptics — particularly those provided by sustained dosing from 'medicated' dressings. The risk assessment for surgical wounds has been defined by the US Study of the Effect of Nosocomial Infection Control (SENIC; Haley *et al*, 1985). This, and other factors has been summarised and put into a continuum by Kingsley (2001a), and revised in this chapter (*Figure 2.2*).

Discussion

Antimicrobial agents have been applied to wounds for thousands of years (Moellering, 1995), but the relentless emergence of resistant strains has forced the continued search for novel agents. As each new type of antibiotic agent has been introduced into clinical practice, changes in microbial sensitivity have been observed. At the outset, there are always some strains that are not inhibited by a new agent (ie. possess intrinsic resistance), and some species that are susceptible. Use of a new antimicrobial agent limits the growth of susceptible strains, but eventually resistant strains always emerge. These agents do not induce the formation of resistance genes, but merely provide an environment in which sensitive species are curtailed and resistant species flourish. Resistance can arise by mutation. It can also arise by the transfer of resistance genes from resistant strains on plasmids or transposons. Cassettes of resistance genes that confer multiple resistance have also been discovered (Collis and Hall, 1995). The emergence of wound pathogens with patterns of multiple antibiotic resistance is having serious consequences in hospital environments (Morgan, 2000), nursing homes (Fraise *et al*, 1997), and the community (Cookson, 2000; Moreno *et al*, 1995). The situation is compounded by the increasing costs of searching for new antimicrobials and the decreasing rate of discovery of new agents.

At one time it was considered that the development of resistance to anti-septics and disinfectants was remote but this has been shown to be incorrect (McDonnell and Russell, 1999). Certain species, such as bacterial endospores, mycobacteria and gram-negative bacteria, possess varying levels of intrinsic resistance, but plasmid-mediated acquired resistance to antiseptics and disinfectants in several bacteria has been reviewed (McDonnell and Russell, 1999). Antiseptics and disinfectants have long been the cornerstone of effective infection control and the prevention of hospital acquired infection. The development of resistance to Triclosan by methicillin resistant *Staphylococcus aureus* is likely to have important consequences for clinical practice.

The presence of different species of micro-organisms in the wound has been linked with delayed healing and wound odour. Trengove and colleagues in Australia (1996) have found a significantly greater chance of impaired healing when four or more species are present. Whilst the definition of wound infection itself is not accepted unanimously (Gilchrist, 1997b; Leaper 1998), the consensus is that the signs are recognised as suppuration, cellulitis, lymphangitis, and bacteraemia. Many texts refer to a figure of 10^5 organisms per gram of tissue as a criterion for infection (Thompson and Smith, 1994). In isolation, this growth density has no confirmed connection to the threshold or degree of immune response, or to healing (Cooper and Lawrence, 1996b); and none at all if no accurate sampling has been conducted (Robson, 1999).

In 'critical' colonisation the numbers of organisms and of species increases above the levels found in the colonised wound. Clinical signs for critical colonisation may be apparent though primarily it is a microbiological criterion that may only become apparent retrospectively once infection is diagnosed. It is possible that delayed healing or the failure to heal in a chronic wound which has no signs of clinical infection, is suggestive of critical colonisation, and is directly related to the microbial bioburden, notably β haemolytic streptococci and anaerobes (Halbert *et al*, 1992). In this study, the implications for wounds colonised with these organisms were that they had been present for longer, were larger, and had a significantly delayed healing time. The implication of these findings being that early, appropriate intervention can avoid progression to critical colonisation and to infection, potentially improving healing rates and reducing the risk of cross infection. Where overt infection exists, systemic antibiotics are usually appropriate first line treatment with topical treatments being useful adjuncts, particularly in the case of poor perfusion. Non-healing wounds where critical colonisation is suspected or confirmed may also be appropriate for topical antibacterial treatment. In the case of silver as an antiseptic, the antibacterial action and effects on indolent wounds (Demling and De Santi, 2001) and burns (Wright *et al*, 1999) have been established. It has been stated that silver can 'provide a disinfected surface in the immediate environment of the wound, thus preventing bacterial infection' (Gilchrist 1996, cited in Williams, 1997). For iodine as iodophor or cadexomer preparations, the consensus is in favour of its use in non-healing and infected chronic wounds (Gilchrist, 1997a; Sundberg and Meller, 1997). Once the infection or critical colonisation is reduced and the wound shows signs of healing, it is advisable to change the dressing for one appropriate to the needs of the wound.

The use of topical silver and iodine containing sustained release formulations on infected and critically colonised wounds can, as part of a holistic approach, be supported. The indications for use of a topical antiseptic sustained delivery system, whether it be dressing, cream or ointment, are several: if one or more overt signs of infection, or any less obvious signs such as increased exudate levels, increased local pain, or cessation of progress in healing occur, then intervention is indicated to return the wound to health. Appropriate topical products will also assist in the reduction of odour and local bioburden, thus reducing the risks of cross infection.

Key points

* Assess all wounds at each dressing change and position them according to the infection continuum.

* Where wounds are static, or exudate levels high, suspect critical colonisation and infection.

* Cleanse, as appropriate, with tap water or saline to remove pus, and tissue and dressing debris.

* Rinsing wounds with antiseptic solutions is of no proven clinical value.

* Pre-treatment of the skin with appropriate antiseptics is effective in reducing the risk of surgical wound infection.

* Topical antibiotics are of very limited value in treating infected wounds; use them with great caution and only where there is no alternative. Systemic antibiotics, dosed appropriately, are indicated for overt infection with signs of spreading cellulitis.

* Dressings and other delivery systems that deliver sustained doses of effective antimicrobials such as silver and iodine have been shown to be valuable in the treatment of critical colonisation and infection.

* Certain dressings can be useful as part of the infection control process.

References

Adams AP, Santschi EM, Mellencamp MA (1999) Antibacterial properties of a silver chloride-coated nylon wound dressing. *Vet Surg* **28**: 219–25
Alinovi A, Bassissi P, Pini M (1986) Systemic administration of antibiotics in the management of venous ulcers. *J Am Acad Dermatol* **15**: 186–91
Ayton M (1985) Wounds that won't heal. *Nurs Times* **81**(46):16–19
Bendy RH, Nuccio PA, Wolfe E *et al* (1964) Relationship of quantitative bacterial counts to healing of decubiti. *Antimicrob Agents Chemother* **4**: 147–55
Bishop JB, Phillips LG, Mustoe TA *et al* (1992) A prospective randomised evaluator-blinded trial of two potential wound healing agents for the treatment of venous stasis ulcers. *J Vasc Surg* **16**: 251–7

Bornier C, Jeannin C (1989) Clinical trials with ACTISORB (Etude clinique Actisorb. Realisee sur 20 cas plaies complexes). *Soins Chir* **99**: 39–41

Bornside GH, Bornside BB (1979) Comparison between moist swab and tissue biopsy methods for bacteria in experimental incision wounds. *J Trauma* **19**: 103–5

Bowler PG, Davies BJ (1999) The microbiology of acute and chronic wounds. *Wounds* **11**: 72–9

Bowler PG, Delargy H, Prince D, Fondberg L (1993) The viral barrier properties of some wound dressings and their role in infection control. *Wounds* **5**: 1–8

Bowler PG, Jones SA, Davies BJ, Coyle E (1999a) Infection control properties of some wound dressings. *J Wound Care* **8**(10): 499–502

Bowler PG, Davies BJ, Jones SA (1999b) Microbial involvement in chronic wound malodour. *J Wound Care* **8**(10): 216–8

Bowler PG, Jones SA, Holland A (2000) *Is silver incorporated into activated charcoal cloth likely to be tough on wound infection?* Poster presentation: Wounds 2000, Harrogate, 12–14 Nov

Bowler PG, Duerden BI, Armstrong DG (2001) Wound microbiology and associated approaches to wound management. *Clin Micro Rev* **14**(2): 244–69

Brennan SS, Leaper DJ (1985) The effect of antiseptics on the healing wound. *Br J Surg* **72**: 780–2

British Medical Journal (1977) Topical antibiotics (Anonymous Editorial). *Br Med J* **1**: 494

Buckley SC, Scott K, Das K (2000) Late review of the use of silver sulphadiazine dressing for the treatment of fingertip injuries. *Injury* **31**(5): 301–4

Bucknall TE (1980) The effect of local infection upon wound healing: an experimental study. *Br J Surg* **67**: 851–5

Burks RI (1998) Povidone-iodine solution in wound treatment. *Phys Ther* **78**: 212–8

Cassino R, Ricci E, Carusone A (2001) *Management of Infected Wounds: a review of antibiotic and antiseptic treatments*. Poster presentation European Wound Management Association, Dublin, 17–19 May

Cervantes C, Silver S (1996) Metal resistance in pseudomonas; genes and mechanisms. In: Nakazawa T, Furakawa K, Haas D, Silver S, eds. *Molecular Biology of Pseudomonads*. American Society for Microbiology,Washington DC, USA

Collis CM, Hall RM (1995) Expression of antibiotic resistance genes in the integrated cassettes of intergrons. *Antimicrobial Agents and Chemotherapy* **39**: 155–62

Colsky AS, Kisner R, Kerdel F (1998) Analysis of antibiotic susceptibilities of skin flora in hospitalised dermatology patients. The crisis of antibiotic resistance has come to the surface. *Arch Dermatol* **134**: 1006–9

Cookson BD (2000) Methicillin-resistant Staphylococcus aureus in the community: New battlefronts, or are the battles lost? *Infect Control Hosp Epidemiol* **21**(6): 398–403

Cooper R, Lawrence JC (1996a) Microorganisms and wounds. *J Wound Care* **5**(5): 233–6

Cooper R, Lawrence JC (1996b) The prevalence of bacteria and implications for infection control. *J Wound Care* **5**(6): 291–5

Cooper R, Molan P (1999) The use of honey as an antiseptic in managing Pseudomonas infections. *J Wound Care* **8**(4): 161–4

Cooper R, Molan P, Harding KG (1999) Antibacterial activity of honey against strains of *Staphylococcus aureus* from infected wounds. *J Roy Soc Med* **92**: 283–5

Cooper R, Molan PC, Krishnamoorthy L, Harding KG (2001) Manuka honey used to heal a recalcitrant surgical wound. *Eur J Clin Micro Inf Dis* **20**: 758–9

Cutting KF, Harding KG (1994) Criteria for identifying wound infection. *J Wound Care* **3**(4): 198–201

Cutting KF (1999) The causes and prevention of maceration of the skin. *J Wound Care* **8**(4): 200–2

Dale JJ, Callam MJ, Ruckley CV, Harper DR, Berry PN (1983) Chronic ulcers of the leg: a study of prevalence in a Scottish community. *Health Bull* **41**: 310–14

Daltrey DC, Rhodes B, Chattwood JG (1981) Investigation into the microbial flora of healing and non-healing decubitus ulcers. *J Clin Pathol* **34**: 701–5

de Haan BB, Ellis H, Wilks M (1974) The role of infection on wound healing. *Surg Gynecol Obstet* **138**: 693–700

DeMarini DM, Brock KH, Doerr CL, Moore MM (1988) Mutagenicity and clastogenicity of proflavin in L5178Y/TK cells. *J Mutat Res* **204**(2): 323–8

Demling RH, DeSanti L (2001) The role of silver in wound healing. Part 1: Effects of silver on wound management. *Wounds* **13**(1) Suppl A3–A15

Drug and Therapeutics Bulletin (1991) Local applications to wounds: 1. Cleansers, antibacterials, debriders. *Drug Ther Bull* **29**(24): 93–5

Duerden BI (1994) Virulence factors in anaerobes. *Clin Infect Dis* **18** (Suppl): S253–S259

Dunford C, Cooper R, Molan P, White RJ (2000) The use of honey in wound management. *Nurs Standard* **15**(11): 63–8

Elek SD (1956) Experimental staphylococcal infections in the skin of man. *Ann NY Acad Sci* **65**: 85–90

Emmerson M (1998) A microbiologist's view of factors contributing to infection. *New Horizons* **6**(2): Suppl S3–S10

Eriksson G, Eklund A-E, Kallings LO (1984) The clinical significance of bacterial growth in venous leg ulcers. *Scand J Infect Dis* **16**: 175–80

Federal Register (1994) Topical antimicrobial drug products for over the counter human use; tentative final monograph for health care antiseptic drug products. *Federal Register* **58**(116): 17 June

Fraise AP, Mitchell K, O'Brien SJ *et al* (1997) Methicillin-resistant Staphylococcus aureus in nursing homes in a major UK city: an anonymised point prevalence study. *Epidemiol Infect* **118**: 1–5

Furr JR, Russell AD, Turner TD, Andrews A (1994) Antibacterial activity of Actisorb Plus, Actisorb and silver nitrate. *J Hosp Infect* **27**: 201–8

Gilchrist B (1997a) Should iodine be reconsidered in wound management? *J Wound Care* **6**(3): 148–50

Gilchrist B (1997b) Wound Infection. In: M Miller, D Glover, eds. *Wound Management*. NT Books, London

Goldenheim PD (1993) An appraisal of povidone-iodine and wound healing. *Postgrad Med J* **69**(Suppl): S97–S105

Gilman A, Rall TW, Nies AS, Taylor P, eds (1990) *Goodman and Gilman's The Pharmacological Basis of Therapeutics 1990*. 8th edn. Pergamon, New York: chap 45, 'Antimicrobials'

Gulliver G (1999) Arguments over iodine. *Nurs Times* **95**(27): 68–70

Gupta R, Foster ME, Miller E (1991) Calcium alginate in the management of acute surgical wounds and abscesses. *J Tissue Viabil* **1**(4): 115–6

Halbert AR, Stacey MC, Rohr JB, Jopp-McKay A (1992) The effect of bacterial colonisation on venous ulcer healing. *Aust J Dermatol* **33**: 75–80

Hansson C, Faergemann J (1995) The effect of antiseptic solutions on micro-organisms in venous leg ulcers. *Acta Derm Venereol* (Stockh) **75**: 31–3

Haley RW, Culver DH, Morgan WM *et al* (1985) Identifying patients at high risk of surgical wound infection: A simple multivariate index of patient susceptibility and wound contamination. *Am J Epidemiol* **121**: 206–15

Hall Angeras M, Brandberg A, Falk A, Seeman T (1992) Comparison between sterile saline and tap water for the acute traumatic soft tissue wounds. *Eur J Surg* **158**: 147–50

Hansis M (1996) Pathophysiology of infection — a theoretical approach. *Injury* **27**: C5–C8

Haughton W, Young T (1995) Common problems in wound care: malodorous wounds. *Br J Nurs* **4**(16): 959–63

Hepburn HH (1919) Delayed primary suture of wounds. *Br Med J* **1**: 181–3

Hunt TK, Hopf HW (1997) Wound healing and wound infection. What surgeons and anaesthesiologists can do. *Surg Clin North Am* **77**(3): 587–606

Huovinen S, Kotilainen P, Jarvinen H *et al* (1994) Comparison of ciprofloxacin or trimethoprim therapy for venous leg ulcers: results of a pilot study. *J Am Acad Dermatol* **31**: 279–81

Hunt TK (1981) Surgical wound infections: an overview. *Am J Med* **70**: 712–18

Hutchinson JJ, Lawrence JC (1991) Wound infection under occlusive dressings. *J Hosp Infect* **17**: 83–94

Iwamoto Y, Ferguson LR, Pearson A, Baguley BC (1992) Photo-enhancement of the mutagenicity of 9-anilinoacridine derivatives related to the antitumour agent amsacrine. *J Mutat Res* **268**(1): 35–41

Jackson DM, Lowbury EJL, Topley E (1951) Chemotherapy of streptococcus infection in burns. *Lancet* **2**: 705–11

Jones R (2001) Honey and healing through the ages. In: Munn P, Jones R, eds. *Honey & Healing*. Ibra, Cardiff

Kaye ET (2000) Topical antibacterial agents. *Infect Dis Clin North Am* **14**(2): 321–39

Kingsley A (2001a) Wound infection and guidelines for effective resolution. *Nurs Standard* **15**(30): 50–8

Kingsley A (2001b) The use of honey in the treatment of infected wounds: case studies. *Br J Nurs* **10**(22): S13–S20

Kramer SA (1999) Effect of povidone-iodine on wound healing: A review. *J Vasc Nurs* **XVII**(1): 17–23

Krizek TJ, Robson MC, Kho E (1967) Bacterial growth and skin graft survival. *Surg Forum* **18**: 518–9

Lawrence JC (1998a) The use of iodine as an antiseptic agent. *J Wound Care* **7**(8): 421–5

Lawrence JC (1998b) A povidone-iodine medicated dressing. *J Wound Care* **7**(7): 332–6

Lawrence JC, Lilly HA, Kidson A (1992) Wound dressings and airborne dispersal of bacteria. *Lancet* **339**: 807

Lawrence JC (1994) Dressings and wound infection. *Am J Surg* **167**(1A): 21S–24S

Leaper DJ (1988) Antiseptic toxicity in open wounds. *Nurs Times* **84**(25): 77–9

Leaper DJ (1992) Eusol. *Br Med J* **304**: 930–1

Leaper DJ (1994) Prophylactic and therapeutic role of antibiotics in wound care. *Am J Surg* **167**(1A): 15S–19S

Leaper DJ (1998) Defining infection (editorial). *J Wound Care* **7**(8): 373.

Lookingbill DP, Miller SH, Knowles RC (1978) Bacteriology of chronic leg ulcers. *Arch Dermatol* **114**: 1765–8

Lyczak JB, Cannon CL, Pier GB (2000) Pseudomonas aeruginosa infection: lessons from a versatile opportunist. *Microbes Infect* **2**(9): 1051–60

Madsen SM, Westh H, Danielsen L, Rosdahl VT (1996) Bacterial colonization and healing of venous leg ulcers. *APMIS* **104**: 895–9

Mangram AJ *et al* (1999) Guidelines for the prevention of surgical site infection. *Am J Infect Control* **27**(2): 97–132

McDonnell G, Russell AD (1999) Antiseptics and disinfectants: activity, action and resistance. *Clin Microbiol Rev* **12**(1): 147–79

McLure AR, Gordon J (1992) In vitro evaluation of povidone-iodine and chlorhexidine against methicillin-resistant Staphylococcus aureus. *J Hosp Infect* **21**: 291–9

Mertz PM, Oliviera-Gandia MF, Davis S (1999) The evaluation of a cadexomer iodine wound dressing on methicillin resistant Staphylococcus aureus (MRSA) in acute wounds. *Dermatol Surg* **25**(2): 89–93

Millward P (1991) Comparing treatments for leg ulcers. *Nurs Times* **87**(13): 70–2

Modak SM, Fox CL (1981) Sulfadiazine silver-resistant Pseudomonas in burns. *Arch Surg* **116**: 854–7

Moellering RC (1995) Past, present, and future of antimicrobial agents. *Am J Med* **99**(Suppl 6A): 11S–18S

Molan P (1992) The antibacterial activity of honey 1. The nature of the antibacterial activity. *Bee World* **73**(1): 5–28

Molan P (1999) The role of honey in the management of wounds. *J Wound Care* 8(8): 415–18

Moreno F, Crisp C, Jorgensen JH, Patterson JE (1995) MRSA as a community organism. *Clin Infect Dis* **21**(5): 1308–12

Moore D (1992) Hypochlorites: a review of the evidence. *J Wound Care* **1**(4): 44–53

Morgan M (2000) The population impact of MRSA: the national survey of MRSA in Wales 1997. *J Hosp Infect* **44**(3): 227–39

Morison M (1990) Wound cleansing — which solution? *Nurs Standard* **4**(52): 4–6

Natarajan S, Williamson D, Grey J, Harding KG, Cooper RA (2001) Healing of an MRSA-colonized, hydroxy-urea induced leg ulcer with honey. *J Derm Treat* **12**: 33–6

Nichols RL (1998) Post operative infections in the age of drug-resistant Gram positive bacteria. *Am J Med* **104**(5A): 11S–16S

Oliver L (1997) Wound cleansing. *Nurs Standard* **11**(20): 44–51

O'Meara SO, Cullum N, Majid M, Sheldon T (2000) Systematic reviews of wound care management: (3) Antimicrobial agents. *Health Technol Assess* **4**(21): 1–237

O'Meara SO, Cullum N, Majid M, Sheldon T (2001) Systematic review of antimicrobial agents used for chronic wounds. *Br J Surg* **88**: 4–21

Pruitt BA (1987) Opportunistic infections in burn patients: diagnosis and treatment. In: Root R, Trunkey R, Sande MA, eds. *New Surgical and Medical Approaches to Infectious Diseases*. Churchill Livingstone, New York: 245–61

Raahave D, Friis-Moller A, Bjerre-Jespen K, Rasmussen LB (1986) The infective dose of aerobic and anaerobic bacteria in post-operative wound sepsis. *Arch Surg* **121**: 924–9

Raju DR, Jindrak K, Weiner M, Endquist IF (1977) A study of the critical bacterial innoculum to cause a stimulus to wound healing. *Surg Gynecol Obstet* **144**: 347–50

Rice TT (1992) Metronidazole use in malodorous skin lesions. *J Rehab Nurs* **17**(5): 244–55

Robson MC (1999) Lessons gleaned from the sport of wound watching. *Wound Repair Regen* **7**(1): 1–6

Robson M, Heggers JP (1969) Bacterial quantification of open wounds. *Mil Med* **134**: 19–24

Robson MC, Heggers JP (1970) Delayed wound closures based on bacterial counts. *J Surg Oncol* **2**: 379–83

Robson M, Steinberg BD, Heggers JP (1990) Wound healing alterations caused by infection. *Clin Plast Surg* **17**: 485–92

Rodeheaver G (1988) Controversies in topical wound management: wound cleansing and wound disinfection. In: Krasner D, ed. *Chronic Wound Care*. Pennsylvania Health Management Publications, USA

Roe B, Cullum N (1995) The management of leg ulcers: current nursing practice. In: Cullum N, Roe B, eds. *Leg Ulcers: Nursing Management. A Research-based Guide*. Scutari Press, London

Roe BH, Luker KA, Cullum NA, Griffiths JM, Kenrick M (1994) Nursing treatment of patients with chronic leg ulcers in the community: report of a survey. *J Clin Nurs* **3**(3): 159–68

Russell AD, Hugo WB (1994) Antimicrobial activity and action of silver. *Prog Med Chem* **31**: 351–70

Saffle JR, Schnebly WA (1994) Burn wound care. In: Richard RL, Stanley MJ, eds. *Burn Care and Rehabilitation: Principles and Practice*. Davis Co. Philadelphia USA: 137–9

Scanlon E, Dowsett C (2001) Clinical governance in the control of wound infection. *Br J Nurs* **10**(22) (Silver Suppl): 12–18

Schraibman IG (1990) The significance of β-haemolytic streptococci in chronic leg ulcers. *Ann Royal Coll Surg Eng* **72**: 123–4

Scott Ward R, Saffle JR (1995) Topical agents in burn wound care. *Phys Ther* **75**(6): 526–38

Scottish Intercollegiate Guidelines Network (1998) *The Care of Patients with Chronic Leg Ulcer. A National Clinical Guideline*. Royal College of Physicians, Edinburgh www.show.cee.hw.ac.uk/sign/home.htm

Selwyn S (1981) The topical treatment of skin infections. In: Maibach H, Aly R, eds. *Skin Microbiology: Relevance to Clinical Infection*. Springer Verlag, New York

Sundberg J, Meller R (1997) A retrospective review of the use of cadexomer iodine in the treatment of chronic wounds. *Wounds* **9**(3): 68–86

Tamuzzer RW, Schultz GS (1996) Biochemical analysis of acute and chronic wound environments. *Wound Rep Regen* **4**: 411–20

Tebbe B, Orfanos CE (1996) Therapy of leg ulcers and decubitus ulcers with a Xerodressing: Modern wound dressing with antibacterial activity. *H+G Band* **71**(9): 697–702

Tenorio A, Jindrak K, Weiner M (1976) Accelerated healing in infected wounds. *Surg Gynecol Obstet* **142**: 537–43

Teplitz C, Davis D, Mason AD, Moncrief JA (1964) *Pseudomonas aeruginosa* burn wound sepsis. *J Surg Res* **4**: 200–16

Thomas C (1988) Nursing alert — wound healing halted with the use of povidone-iodine. *Ostomy/Wound Management* **18**(Spring): 30–33

Thomas S, Fisher B, Fram PJ, Waring MJ (1998a) Odour-absorbing dressings. *J Wound Care* **7**(5): 246–50

Thomas S, Fisher B, Fram PJ, Waring MJ (1998b) Odour-absorbing dressings. www.smtl.co.uk/World-Wide-Wounds/1998/march/odour-absorbing-dressings.htm

Thomlinson D (1997) To clean or not to clean? *Nurs Times* **83**(9): 71–5

Thompson PD, Smith DJ (1994) What is infection? *Am J Surg* **167** (1A) (Suppl): 7S–11S

Tonks A, Cooper RA, Price AJ, Molan PC, Jones KP (2001) Stimulation TNFα release in monocytes by honey. *Cytokine* **14**(4): 240–2

Trengove N, Stacey M, McGechie D *et al* (1996) Qualitative bacteriology and leg ulcer healing. *J Wound Care* **5**(6): 277–80

White RJ (2001) A charcoal dressing with silver in wound infection; clinical evidence. *Br J Nurs* **10**(22) (Silver suppl): 4–11

White RJ, Cooper R, Kingsley A (2001) Wound colonization and infection: the role of topical antimicrobials. *Br J Nurs* **10**(9): 563–78

Williams C (1994) Actisorb Plus in the treatment of exuding infected wounds. *Br J Nurs* **3**(15): 786–8

Williams C (1997) Arglaes controlled release dressing in the control of bacteria. *Br J Nurs* **6**(2): 114–15

Willix D, Molan P, Harfoot C (1992) A comparison of the sensitivity of wound-infecting species of bacteria to the antibacterial activity of manuka honey and other honey. *J Appl Bacteriol* **73**: 388–94

Wright JB, Lam K, Burrell RE (1998a) Wound management in an era of increasing bacterial antibiotic resistance: A role for topical silver treatment. *Am J Infect Control* **26**(6): 572–7

Wright JB, Hansen DL, Burrell RE (1998b) The comparative efficacy of two antimicrobial barrier dressings: in vitro examination of two controlled release silver dressings. *Wounds* **10**: 179–88

Wright JB, Lam K, Hansen DL, Burrell RE (1999) Efficacy of topical silver against fungal burn wound pathogens. *Am J Infect Control* **27**(4): 344–50

Wunderlich U, Orfanos CE (1991) Treatment of venous leg ulcers with silver-impregnated xero-dressings. *Hautartz* **42**: 446–50

Yin HQ, Langford R, Burrell RE (1999) Comparative evaluation of Acticoat antimicrobial barrier dressing. *J Burn Care Rehab* **20**: 195–200

Zaki I, Shall L, Dalziel KL (1994) Bacitracin: a significant sensitiser in leg ulcer patients? *Contact Dermatitis* **31**: 92–94

3

Applying the principles of infection control to wound care

Lynn Parker

Human skin in healthy adults is inhospitable to pathogenic organisms. A wound may occur from any accidental or deliberate trauma that breaks the surface of the skin. Once this line of defence is broken there is a risk of infection. All soft tissue injuries, whether chronic, traumatic or surgical, involve the same basic biochemical and cellular processes. This chapter looks at the risk factors associated with healing of such wounds. The principles of asepsis, wound cleansing agents, choice of dressings and the taking of wound swabs are considered.

The first line of defence against infection is the skin (*Figure 3.1*); any wound that disrupts this line of defence creates a risk of infection. In a broad sense, wounds may occur from any accidental or deliberate trauma that breaks the surface of the skin or mucous membranes. This includes pressure sores and leg ulcers caused by vascular or neural pathology. The entry points of drainage tubes and wires into body cavities and the cardiovascular system are also included as wounds.

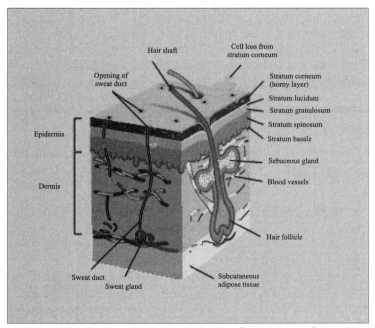

Figure 3.1: Diagrammatic representation of the layers of the skin

Human skin in healthy adults is inhospitable to pathogenic organisms. Bacteria are the most common inhabitants of the skin especially Gram-positive organisms such as *Staphylococcus epidermidis* and diphtheroid. Resident flora live on or in the superficial layers of the epidermal stratum corneum and also in the upper parts of the sweat glands and hair follicles. They are found all over the body but the highest numbers are found in the scalp and moist areas of the body. The majority are generally harmless but have the ability to become pathogenic if they penetrate the skin through surgical procedures or the insertion of invasive devices.

Other organisms can be transient in nature and do not multiply on healthy skin. They are usually acquired from other sites on the body, from another person, or from the environment. Transient organisms include *Staphylococcus aureus* which colonises the anterior nares and the perineal area in 20% of healthy people (Lowbury *et al*, 1992) but may be temporarily transferred to other areas of the skin. Skin cells are continually being shed from the surface of the body and bacteria are dispersed on them with *Staphylococcus aureus* being the most common organism associated with dispersal. If a person has any skin disease, such as psoriasis, where the epidermal turnover rate is increased, the number of organisms dispersed is increased (Shanson, 1999).

Gram-negative organisms, such as *Escherichia coli* and *Pseudomonas* spp., are also acquired transiently on the skin, especially the hands. They survive for several hours unless effectively removed by good hand washing. Additional problems can occur when anaerobic organisms like *Clostridium perfringens*, found in the gastrointestinal tract, colonise the skin around the thighs and buttocks especially in elderly patients confined to bed. Careful preparation of the skin is essential before orthopaedic surgery of the lower limbs.

It is important to remember that the skin provides both a mechanical and chemical barrier to organisms; organisms cannot penetrate the horny keratin layer of the skin if it is unbroken. Acidity and fatty acid content from the skin's secretions are bactericidal like the antimicrobial substances produced by flora resident on the skin. So, the normal flora of the skin plays a vital role in maintaining a microbial balance that if disrupted can lead to invasion by opportunistic or pathogenic organisms which will create an imbalance in the system.

Types of wounds

The same basic biochemical and cellular processes are involved in the healing of all soft-tissue injuries, whether they are the chronic ulcerative wounds of leg ulcers and pressure sores, or the traumatic wounds of lacerations, abrasions and burns, and surgical wounds.

Wound healing can be classified into three stages of primary, secondary and tertiary intention (Brunner and Suddarth, 1992) (*Table 3.1*). The risk of a wound acquiring an infection is dependent upon the individual patient's susceptibility to acquiring an infection and the ability of the wound to heal. Such susceptibility includes general risk factors such as underlying disease that may depress the response of the immune system (Wilson, 1995). Correlation exists between increasing age and the risk of developing a wound infection; poor nutrition, weight loss, and obesity are also associated with an increased risk of infection (Cruse and Foord, 1973; Bucknall, 1985).

The physiological changes in the body associated with ageing may lead to a decreased efficiency of the mechanisms that aid wound healing. Over the age of thirty years the body ages at different rates affecting the cardiac and immune systems. Disease of the circulatory system can delay wound healing and with ageing a decrease in the replacement of epidermal cells and a reduced inflammatory response occur (Russell, 2000). Chronic wounds contain large amounts of degrading tissue that can delay wound healing (Wysocki, 1996). Infected wounds have a different exudate than uninfected wounds including bacterial toxins that may indirectly delay wound healing.

Table 3.1: Three stages of wound healing
Primary intention: With wounds that have breaks in the skin caused by trauma or surgical procedures, the edges of the skin are brought together using staples, sutures, or glue, and a fine scar is formed; healing is often quick with minimal scarring
Secondary intention: These wounds extend into the dermis or deeper layers; include chronic and long-standing wounds, such as leg ulcers and pressure sores, and these may become infected
Tertiary intention: These wounds usually occur when a surgical wound has broken down. Surgical intervention is often required to remove the cause of the infection, either a haematoma or large collection of pus, that can cause a wound to dehisce

Russell, 2000

Reducing the temperature of the wound may hinder the activity of certain cells; if the wound temperature drops from the optimum of 37°C to 28°C then leucocyte activity stops (Russell, 2000). Such a drop in temperature may be caused by removing dressings for ward rounds; covering wounds with green towels at this time may also expose them to bacterial contamination. The risk of infection in surgical wounds is dependent on a delicate balance between bacteria present in the wound at the end of the operation and the person's own host immune defence.

Most factors associated with the development of surgical wound infections are outside the control of nurses. The risk is dependent upon the level of contamination at the time of surgery, with the bacteria that cause such wound infections frequently being derived from the patient's own normal flora. The number of bacteria in the wound at the end of the procedure depends upon the site of the body being operated on. Therefore, a system of wound contamination classification as shown in (*Table 3.2*) has been developed.

Table 3.2: Classification of wound contamination

Category	Description	Type of surgery	Approximate infection rate (%)
Clean	Gastrointestinal and respiratory tract not entered. No inflamed tissue, no break in technique	Orthopaedic surgery Neurosurgery	<2
Clean-contaminated	Gastrointestinal or respiratory tract entered but no spillage of contents	Appendicectomy	8
Contaminated	Acute inflamed tissue, spillage from hollow organ, traumatic wounds, major break in technique	Abdominal surgery	15
Dirty	Pus encountered, perforated hollow organ, delayed treatment of traumatic wounds	Drainage of abscess	40

Wilson, 1995

Other factors that influence a patient's risk of contracting an infection following surgery include the length of their preoperative stay. This is thought to be due to two possible reasons (*Table 3.3*).

Table 3.3: Two main reasons for contracting an infection following surgery

Those patients that require an extended stay are probably debilitated or present with a co-existing illness
The preoperative stay may increase contamination of the skin by pathogenic organisms already present in the hospital

Mishriki *et al*, 1992

Preparation of the patient before surgery has identified risk factors of preoperative shaving and bathing. Attempts at trying to reduce the level of colonisation of the skin by patients bathing or showering has been advocated as a means of minimising their risk of infection. The effectiveness of this practice has not been demonstrated in published studies (Ayliffe *et al*, 1983; Lynch *et al*, 1992). A number of studies have shown that shaving the skin before surgery increases the risk of infection, with some studies showing an infection rate of 5.6% in shaved patients as opposed to 1% in unshaven patients or in those in which a depilatory cream was used (Seropian and Reynolds, 1971; Cruse, 1992).

The razor on the surface of the skin causes microabrasions, especially if the patient is shaved many hours before surgery. Use of electric shavers has been associated with a lower infection rate; however, their use presents other problems with respect to the risk of cross-infection (Millward, 1992). A suitable alternative may be the use of hair clippers which cause less damage to the skin (Pettersson, 1986).

Perioperative risk factors for patients include the technique of the surgeon, duration of surgery, ventilation and cleanliness of the theatre environment, and sterility of instruments (Horton and Parker, 1997).

Principles of asepsis

When undertaking wound care the use of aseptic techniques, in which sterile equipment, cleansing agents, dressings and sterile gloves are used, prevents the transmission of microbes to the wound. The aseptic method is frequently advocated in the literature for changing wound dressings and is standard recommended practice (Lund and Caruso, 1993; Horton and Parker, 1997; Hollinworth and Kingston, 1998). An alternative approach is now being advocated that suggests a clean technique may be applicable for certain wounds; here, non-sterile gloves may be worn and certain chronic wounds in some patients may be irrigated using solutions such as tap water (Riyat and Quinton, 1997; Hollinworth and Kingston, 1998)

Handwashing

The aseptic technique is one area of nursing practice in which a ritual can be recognised from when to wash your hands, cleaning of the trolley, opening the dressing pack, to cleaning the wound. The hands of nurses are recognised as a common vehicle for the transfer of microbes between patients and staff. The antibacterial properties of the skin prevent the survival of transient flora for more than a few hours (Wilson, 1995). Many skin-cleansing agents are available but most transient flora are quickly removed by thorough washing with soap and water followed by hand drying. The frequency with which handwashing should be undertaken during wound care depends upon the individual circumstances of the patient's wound. Excessive washing may damage the skin and increase the risk of hand colonisation with pathogens (Ayliffe *et al*, 1992; Gould, 1993).

Gloves

The use of gloves has now replaced sterile forceps in dressing packs; this has had an implication on the optimum time to wash hands during the dressing procedure. Some have recommended that where the wound has healed superficially, as in removing a dressing from a sutured wound after twenty-four hours, if hand washing is performed effectively gloves do not need to be worn (Chrintz *et al*, 1989).

It is still necessary for nurses to wash their hands after wearing gloves in order to remove any bacterial growth that has occurred on the hands under the gloves and because the hands may be contaminated as gloves are removed (Ayliffe *et al*, 1992). Whether non-sterile gloves should replace the use of sterile gloves for wound care is debatable. A number of studies seem to suggest that for routine wound care and changes of dressings, clean non-sterile gloves may be used safely (Rossoff *et al*, 1993; Hollinworth and Kingston, 1998).

Sterile or clean fluids

Traditional wound cleansing has routinely meant that a variety of sterile solutions are used to clean a wound with the purpose of removing any material that may delay it from healing. Routine cleansing of any wound should be questioned as cleansing a wound and drying it afterwards goes against the principles of moist wound healing (Pudner, 1997a). Bathing and showering has been recommended as a suitable method for cleansing sacral and perianal wounds and also for leg ulceration (Bucknole, 1996). Tap water is recommended for cleansing open traumatic wounds in accident and emergency departments (Riyat and Quinton, 1997).

Access to a clean water supply that is regularly monitored is essential and if this is possible and individual patients are assessed for their risk of infection it may be a safe practice to follow (Hollinworth and Kingston, 1998). Using holy water to sprinkle on wounds and dressings is not recommended as *Pseudomonas* spp. and *Escherichia coli* have been isolated from Christian shrines, but it can be autoclaved thus rendering it free from pathogens (Nye, 1996).

Sterile or clean products

Most dressing packs and modern occlusive dressings used today for wound care are commercially prepared and as long as the packaging remains dry and intact the contents should remain sterile (Ayliffe *et al*, 1993). Before being used they should be checked for evidence of damage or moisture and if faulty in this way the pack should be returned to the sterile services department.

Wound cleansing agents

Nurses still routinely practise the cleansing of wounds and this is an important part of assisting the healing process; by cleansing the wound any material that may delay healing is removed. This process can be impeded by the presence of necrotic tissue, excess wound exudate, dressing residue, and metabolic waste on the surface of the wound and can increase the potential for infection (Barr, 1995). Cleansing an infected wound may remove some organisms on the surface but has little effect in cleansing the wound bed and surrounding tissues; most surgical wounds require no cleaning (Pudner, 1997a). There are a number of methods of cleansing wounds, including mechanical swabbing, irrigation, bathing or showering, and the use of wound dressing products (see *Chapter 2*).

Mechanical swabbing using cotton wool balls or gauze is not advised as in most cases this is ineffective and can traumatise the wound. Cotton wool fibres can be left behind in the bed of the wound and can cause an inflammatory response. No matter what method is adopted to mechanically clean the wound few organisms are removed, they are just moved around the wound (Thomlinson, 1987). In sloughy wounds mechanical swabbing may help in removing the sloughy tissue but it is important to avoid traumatising the healthy tissue that surrounds the wound (Pudner, 1997a).

Irrigation has become the preferred method in cleansing wounds as it can loosen debris and excess exudate without traumatising the bed of the wound. The problem of fibres shedding into the wound is removed along with the associated problems when this occurs. If the irrigation fluid is not collected into an appropriate container patients may find the procedure unpleasant leaving them wet and uncomfortable. Nurses must also be aware of the risk of splashback and take appropriate protection against contamination (Oliver, 1997).

The pressure applied by the fluid is very important as too great a pressure is likely to damage the granulation tissue and too little will be ineffective (Pudner, 1997a). It is recommended that a pressure of between 4 and 15 pounds per square inch (psi) is used and that 8 psi can cleanse a wound effectively without causing trauma; this can be achieved by using a 35ml syringe and a 19 gauge needle. If nurses use this method they must be careful that the patient is not accidentally injured with the needle (Pudner, 1997a). Nowadays, there are a variety of prepacked devices available, but care must be taken to avoid contaminating the nozzle with exudate from the wound. Neither should single-use irrigation devices be used for multi-use purposes as there is the potential for cross-infection between patients.

Bathing or showering is a suitable method used for leg ulcers, sacral and perianal wounds; however, organisms found in wounds can easily contaminate the bath water so showering is preferred. Having a bath or shower can be refreshing for patients and also reduce the pain and help to remove the old dressing. Using hydrotherapy or a whirlpool is an aggressive form of bathing that uses the turbulence of the water to dislodge the debris from the wound (Williams, 1999). The prevention of cross-infection must be considered and baths must be cleaned before and after use, and a polythene liner placed in a bucket if it is to be used to wash a client's lower leg.

Some wound dressing products have the ability, especially in the area of necrotic or sloughy wounds, to cleanse the wound. Hydrocolloid dressings rehydrate necrotic or sloughy tissue and so aid debridement by preventing the loss of water vapour from the surface of the skin, thus helping the natural autolytic process. Debrisan and Iodosorb can work as cleansing agents by drawing bacteria and debris into the spaces between the beads and so are removed from the wound when the dressing product is replaced (Pudner, 1997a).

A new initiative is the increased use of 'biosurgery' or larval treatment for infected or necrotic wounds. How the larvae kill bacteria in wounds is not fully understood but it may include the production of natural antibiotic-like agents, modification of the wound pH, and the ingestion and destruction of bacteria as part of the normal feeding processes. It is suggested that the use of larvae should be considered earlier in patients' treatment, especially for clean-up problems, in the case of infected wounds as the use of topical or systemic antimicrobial treatments could be reduced (Thomas *et al*, 1999).

Wound cleansing solutions range from normal saline and tap water to antiseptics and hypochlorites. Current practice has moved away from antiseptics and hypochlorites to normal saline and tap water. This is due to evidence showing that many antiseptics are deactivated in the presence of body fluids and that they do not have the long contact times with the wound surface that are required to be effective against bacterial infection (Ferguson, 1988).

Other studies have shown that applying antiseptics to healing wounds could be detrimental to the healing process (Brennan and Leaper, 1985; Brennan *et al*, 1986). Chlorhexidine is effective against Gram-positive and Gram-negative organisms but has a decreased effect in the presence of blood and pus (Brennan *et al*, 1986). Cetrimide has useful detergent properties but is easily contaminated by bacteria such as *Pseudomonas* spp. Hydrogen peroxide destroys anaerobic bacteria and is inactivated when it comes into contact with organic matter; it is recommended that the wound and surrounding tissue be irrigated with normal saline to avoid the risk of skin irritation (Dealey, 1994).

Povidone-iodine is a broad-spectrum antiseptic. There is debate among clinicians regarding the role of iodine in wound management. Sodium hypo-chlorite preparations, such as EUSOL (Edinburgh Universal Solution of Lime) (Milton) and Chlorasol (SSL), have mild antiseptic properties and are not now recommended (Thomas, 1991). Finally, it is important to remember that a vital component in the creation of the most effective environment for wounds to heal in is the maintenance of the surface temperature of wounds. The cleansing agent considered to be the most appropriate needs to be warmed before being used so that body temperature is maintained at the surface of the wound (Pudner, 1997b).

Choice of dressings

The ultimate aim of wound management is to promote healing by primary intention without infection so that there is minimal scarring and normal function. Conventional dressings are able to prevent access of bacteria to wounds. Surgical wounds with haemostasis do not require protection after twenty-four hours although a dressing may cover the closed wound to protect stitches or clips catching on clothing (Meers *et al*, 1994).

Winter's work is often quoted as establishing the concept of moist wound healing (Winter, 1962). Forty years on, there is a plethora of different types of dressings that can be confusing when trying to decide which to use. Dressings that prevent entry of microbes into the wound and allow normal body defence mechanisms to act are the preferred choice. Many types of products have been developed for the management of wounds; these range from foams, absorbent beads, alginate sheets, and cavity dressings, to hydrocolloid dressings (Russell, 2000). Infection in the wound results in an increased production of exudate and the dressing may then need to be changed for absorbency or antimicrobial properties (Thomas, 1997).

The general acceptance is that dressings should, by whatever method, remove excess fluid from the immediate vicinity of the wound and this is frequently stated as a function of the ideal dressing. Nurses should remember that the state of hydration of a wound normally decreases as the wound progresses towards healing. The choice of dressings may need to be reviewed regularly to consider the changes taking place as the wound heals. There should be continuity and regular evaluation of wounds and dressings, with the dressings used being matched to the patient and wound. As the wound healing process progresses the type of dressing may need to be changed to optimise the condition of the wound (Krasner and Sibbald, 1999).

Dressings can be divided into conventional and advanced categories. Conventional dressings include gauze, non-adherent gauze, and impregnated gauze with topical agents and packing strips. Advanced dressings include the major categories of alginates, collagen, films, foams, hydrocolloids and hydrogels. Within each of the categories there is a wide range of products and such dressings should maintain an ideal moist wound environment by absorbing exudate or donating or maintaining moisture (Krasner and Sibbald, 1999).

When considering selection of a wound dressing it is necessary to think about the factors listed in *Table 3.4*. It is important that the patient can maintain normal activity, especially if we are talking about dressings undertaken in the community outside the hospital setting. If the patient is included in the discussion about the use of the most appropriate dressing for his/her wound then compliance to treatment is greatly enhanced (Miller and Collier, 1996).

Table 3.4: Properties required of a dressing
The ability to absorb exudate *vs* donating or maintaining moisture
Adherence or non-adherence
Occlusion or non-occlusion
Frequency of dressing changes needed
Cost-effectiveness
Patient acceptability and compliance

There is still a distinction between primary and secondary dressings with primary dressings being those that fill or touch the wound and secondary dressings being those that secure the primary dressing. However, many of the advanced dressings can perform either function (Krasner and Sibbald, 1999)

Specimen collection and laboratory reports

Taking a wound swab must be one of the most common specimens collected by nursing staff. The information gained from such specimens can in some instances be questionable, depending upon the quality of the specimen and the information given on the accompanying form. Routine specimens are rarely taken these days and wound swabs should be taken as a result of assessment of the patient's wound and the suspicion that it may be infected.

A wound should show the signs of infection: pus, inflammation, erythema or pyrexia. It must be remembered that a wide range of bacteria can be isolated from a wound swab, but many may just colonise the wound (Wilson, 1995). It is important to remember to treat the patient and not the laboratory report. Accurate information about the patient that is relevant to the specimen should be included, along with any current antibiotics being used, as this will assist the laboratory staff when considering which tests are most appropriate.

In practice, most specimens are taken by swabbing the surface of the wound but this can give misleading information as the results generally reflect bacterial colonisation (Gilchrist, 2000). A sample of pus or tissue is always more useful than a wound swab (Wilson, 1993). It is always worthwhile obtaining advice from the laboratory if you are uncertain as to the type of specimen that needs to be taken. A range of advice is given on taking wound swabs and no definitive method currently exists; there is conflicting information in the literature.

There is debate regarding whether wounds should be cleaned or not before taking the specimen; some authors state that surface contamination should be removed (Cooper and Lawrence, 1996) while others maintain that the swabs need to be taken before cleansing when the maximum number of bacteria are present (Wilson, 1995). A zigzag motion across the surface of the wound rotating the swab between the fingers at the same time, is recommended by the Wound Care Society (Committee Members of the Wound Care Society, 1993). A general preference for using transport medium is recommended, usually Stuart's medium (Gilchrist, 2000).

Conclusion

The normal flora of the skin plays a vital role in maintaining microbial balance that once disrupted can lead to invasion by opportunistic or pathogenic organisms. Wounds may occur from any accidental or deliberate trauma that breaks the surface of the skin or mucous membranes. Once the first line of defence is disrupted it creates a risk of infection. The same biochemical and cellular processes are involved in all types of wounds.

Wound management is individual to each patient and requires that staff understand and apply the principles of asepsis in accordance with current best practice. Staff should be knowledgeable of the wound healing process and the correct dressing to be used depending upon the type of wound. Specimen collection with wound swabs should not be routine but purposeful to help in assessing the type of infection in order to assist in effective antibiotic prescribing.

Key points

❖ The normal flora of the skin plays a vital role in maintaining microbial balance that once disrupted can lead to invasion by opportunistic or pathogenic organisms.

❖ Risk of wounds to acquire an infection is dependent upon an individual patient's susceptibility to acquire an infection and the ability of the wound to heal.

❖ Wound swabs should not be taken routinely but used only to assess the cause of infection and influence effective antibiotic prescribing.

❖ Modern advanced wound dressings maintain the ideal moist wound environment for healing.

❖ Staff should be knowledgeable of the wound healing process and the correct dressing to be used according to the type of wound.

References

Ayliffe GAJ, Noy ME, Davies JG *et al* (1983) A comparison of preoperative bathing with chlorhexidine detergent and a non-medicated soap in the prevention of wound infection. *J Hosp Infection* **4**: 237–44

Ayliffe GAJ, Lowbury EJL, Geddes AM, Williams JD (1992) *Control of Hospital Infection: A Practical Handbook*. 3rd edn. Chapman and Hall, London

Ayliffe GAJ, Collins BJ, Taylor LJ (1993) *Hospital-acquired Infection. Principles and Prevention*. 2nd edn. Butterworth-Heinemann, Oxford

Barr JE (1995) Principles of wound cleansing. *Ostomy/Wound Man* **41**(Suppl 7A): 15–21

Brennan S, Leaper D (1985) The effect of antiseptics on the healing wound: a study using the rabbit ear chamber. *Br J Surg* **72**: 780–2

Brennan S, Foster M, Leaper D (1986) Antiseptic toxicity in wound healing by secondary intention. *J Hosp Infection* **8**: 263–7

Brunner L, Suddarth D (1992) *Textbook of Adult Nursing*. Chapman and Hall, London

Bucknall TE (1985) Factors affecting the development of surgical wound infections: a surgeon's view. *J Hosp Infection* **6**: 1–8

Bucknole W (1996) Treating venous ulcers in the community. *J Wound Care* **5**(5): 258–60

Chrintz H, Vibits H, Cordtz TO *et al* (1989) Need for surgical wound dressing. *Br J Surg* **76**: 204–5

Collier M (1996) The principles of optimum wound management. *Nurs Standard* **10**(43): 47–52

Committee Members of the Wound Care Society (1993) Wound swab procedure. *J Wound Care* **2**(2): 77

Cooper R, Lawrence JC (1996) The isolation and identification of bacteria from wounds. *J Wound Care* **5**(7): 335–40

Cruse PJE (1992) Classification of operations and audit of infection. In: Taylor EW, ed. *Infection in Surgical Practice*. Oxford University Press, Oxford

Cruse PJE, Foord R (1973) A five-year prospective study of 23 649 surgical wounds. *Arch Surg* **107**: 206

Dealey C (1994) *The Care of Wounds*. Blackwell Scientific Publications, Oxford

Ferguson A (1988) Best performer. *Nurs Times* **84**(14): 52–5

Gilchrist B (2000) Taking a wound swab. *Nurs Times* **96**(4): 2

Gould D (1993) Assessing nurses' hand decontamination performance. *Nurs Times* **89**(25): 47–50

Hollinworth H, Kingston JE (1998) Using a non-sterile technique in wound care. *Prof Nurse* **13**(4): 226–9

Horton R, Parker L (1997) *Informed Infection Control Practice*. Churchill Livingstone, New York

Krasner DL, Sibbald RG (1999) Nursing management of chronic wounds. *Nurs Clin North Am* **34**(4): 933–55

Lowbury EJL, Ayliffe GAJ, Geddes AM, Williams JD, eds (1992) *Control of Hospital Infection: A Practical Handbook*. 3rd edn. Chapman and Hall, London

Lund C, Caruso R (1993) Nursing perspectives: aseptic techniques in wound care. *Dermatol Nurs* **5**(3): 215–6

Lynch W, Davey PG, Malek M *et al* (1992) Cost-effectiveness analysis of the use of chlorhexidine detergent in preoperative whole-body disinfection in wound infection prophylaxis. *J Hosp Infection* **21**: 179–91

Meers P, Jackson W, McPherson M (1994) *Hospital Infection Control for Nurses*. Chapman and Hall, New York

Miller M, Collier M (1996) Understanding wounds. *Professional Nurse* (supplement). In association with Johnson & Johnson Medical, EMAP Healthcare, London

Millward S (1992) The hazards of communal razors. *Nurs Times* **88**(6): 58–62

Mishriki SF, Jeffrey PJ, Law DJW (1992) Wound infection: the surgeon's responsibility. *J Wound Care* **1**(2): 32–6

Nye K (1996) Holy water: a risk factor for hospital acquired-infection. *J Hosp Infection* (letter) **33**: 301

Oliver L (1997) Wound cleansing. *Nurs Standard* **20**(11): 47–51

Pettersson E (1986) A cut above the rest? *Nurs Times* **31**(5): 68–70

Pudner R (1997a) Wound cleansing. *J Comm Nurs* **11**(7): 30–6

Pudner R (1997b) Factors affecting the healing process. *J Comm Nurs* **11**(3): 20–6

Riyat MS, Quinton DN (1997) Tap water as a wound cleansing agent in accident and emergency. *J Acc Emerg Med* **14**: 165–6

Rossoff LJ, Lam S, Hilton E *et al* (1993) Is the use of boxed gloves in an intensive care unit safe? *Am J Med* **94**(6): 602–7

Russell L (2000) Understanding physiology of wound healing and how dressings help. *Br J Nurs* **9**(1): 10–21

Seropian R, Reynolds BM (1971) Wound infections after preoperative depilatory *versus* razor preparation. *Am J Surg* **121**: 251–6

Shanson DC (1999) *Microbiology in Clinical Practice*. 3rd edn. Wright, London

Thomas S (1991) Evidence fails to justify use of hypochlorite. *J Tissue Viabil* **1**(1): 9–10

Thomas S (1997) Assessment and management of wound exudate. *J Wound Care* **6**(7): 327–30

Thomas S, Andrews A, Jones M, Church J (1999) Maggots are useful in treating infected or necrotic wounds. *Br Med J* **318**: 807

Thomlinson D (1987) To clean or not to clean? *Nurs Times* **83**(9): 71–5

Williams C (1999) Wound irrigation techniques: new Steripod normal saline. *Br J Nurs* **8**(21): 1460–2

Wilson P (1993) Preparing wound samples for analysis. *J Wound Care* **2**(4): 193

Wilson J (1995) *Infection Control in Clinical Practice*. Baillière Tindall, London

Winter G (1962) Formation of the scab and the rate of epithelialization of superficial wounds in the skin of the young domestic pig. *Nature* **193**: 293–4

Wysocki AB (1996) Wound fluids and the pathogenesis of chronic wounds. *J Wound Ostomy Continence Nurse* **23**: 283–90

Section II:
Chronic wounds

4

Investigations in the management of lower limb ulceration

Peter Vowden, Kathryn Vowden

The management of lower limb ulceration must be founded on accurate assessment of the patient, the limb and the ulcer. This chapter explores the varied assessment methods needed to assess fully a patient with lower limb ulceration and emphasises how these aid in establishing the aetiology of an ulcer, the identification of associated risk factors for delayed healing and the selection of appropriate treatment modalities. The chapter also indicates that assessment is an ongoing process recognising that for leg ulceration, as with all chronic diseases, the background health state may change with time and that this may require modification of any treatment plan.

The effective treatment of lower limb ulceration is highly dependent upon establishing the aetiology of the wound and the identification of other associated conditions that may have an adverse effect on healing. Epidemiological studies have provided data on the important diagnostic groupings and the likelihood of many ulcers, particularly in the elderly, having multiple contributory factors. Only by structured and thorough assessment and appropriate investigation can these be identified.

Epidemiological studies have consistently shown that vascular disease and, in particular, venous disease accounts for the majority of lower limb ulcers (Callam *et al*, 1985; Cornwall *et al*, 1986; Lees *et al*, 1992; Baker *et al*, 1994; Nelzen *et al*, 1994). In Western populations up to 70% of patients have venous disease as the predominant factor causing their leg ulceration (Browse and Burnand, 1982).

The next most common aetiological factor is peripheral arterial disease. This becomes an increasingly common contributory factor in the elderly. Cornwall (1986) found that more than 50% of the population over the age of 80 had concomitant arterial disease. In almost 20% of all patients arterial disease will complicate venous ulceration and may therefore affect treatment and healing (Ghauri *et al*, 1998a; Moffatt, 2001). These ulcers are often inappropriately referred to as mixed ulcers for the aetiology of the ulcer itself is rarely mixed (Vowden *et al*, 2001a). Once the likely aetiology of an ulcer has been established one of the primary aims of screening investigations in patients with lower limb ulceration is to exclude significant peripheral arterial disease which may impact on the treatment of any lower limb wound or ulcer.

The diagnosis of a venous ulcer remains a diagnosis of exclusion, based on the presence of venous disease and the exclusion of other causes of ulceration. There is a marked variation in the percentages of non-vascular ulcers present in published series. This probably reflects the clinical specialty involved and the patient numbers. In most series the more unusual causes account for 5–10% of ulcers (Morison and Moffatt, 1994; Salaman and Harding, 1995). These more unusual ulcers may easily be misdiagnosed as venous ulcers if the assessment process is inadequate. Moffatt (2001) has recently reviewed the more unusual causes of leg ulceration which include skin malignancies, blood disorders, infection, metabolic disorders, lymphoedema, iatrogenic and self-inflicted ulceration.

Even with thorough assessment, there remains a small number of ulcers in which no obvious aetiological factor can be identified. In our experience this may account for a further 5–10% of leg ulcers, a finding supported by others (Grabs *et al*, 1996; Guest *et al*, 1999a). These ulcers are frequently initially classified as venous but on investigation with Doppler and duplex ultrasound the limb is found to demonstrate no functional deep or superficial venous reflux. Bjellerup (1997) suggested the term 'hydrostatic ulcers' for some of these wounds.

The UK guidelines for leg ulcer management (RCN Institute, 1998; SIGN, 1998) suggest a framework for the assessment of a patient with a leg ulcer including history, physical examination and Doppler ankle brachial pressure index (ABPI) calculation. Five key areas of patient assessment (*Box 4.1*) are required in the majority of patients before the instigation of treatment and these should identify those factors which may give rise to complications in patients with leg ulceration (*Table 4.1*). While there are undoubted benefits to high compression therapy in the management of venous ulceration, such therapy is not without risks (Callam *et al*, 1987). Even low levels of compression, if used inappropriately, can cause skin damage (Vowden and Vowden, 1996). All patients with a leg ulcer must be fully assessed before compression therapy is instigated (Moffatt, 1993).

When faced with a leg ulcer the assessment process, including any appropriate investigations, should identify:

1. The aetiology of this ulcer.
2. Factors likely to delay healing.
3. The most appropriate treatment taking, for example, the patient's social and physical characteristics into consideration.
4. Correctable risk factors which will speed healing and reduce the risk of ulcer recurrence.

Box 4.1: Key areas in patient assessment	
The patient	History, risk factors, associated disease, build, nutrition, social circumstances, psychological state
The skin	Colour, pigmentation, temperature, cellulitis, sensitivity, fragility/ trauma, liposclerosis, atrophie blanche
The circulation	Pulses, ABPI*, capillary return, venous flare, varicose veins
The limb	Oedema, shape, ankle mobility, patient mobility
The ulcer	Site, size, surface, edge, duration, infection, exudate, pain
*ABPI = ankle brachial pressure index	

Venous disease and venous leg ulceration

Both superficial and deep venous insufficiency produce varying degrees of chronic venous hypertension. Valvular reflux that produces dermal capillary bed damage and alterations in the skin micro-circulation predispose to lower limb ulceration. A number of theories exist as to how these changes produce skin damage (Browse and Burnand, 1982; Coleridge Smith *et al*, 1988; Chant, 1990; Higley *et al*, 1995). Chronic venous hypertension may result in a number of characteristic visible changes in the limb and skin, particularly in the gaiter area. These include skin staining, lipodermatosclerosis, atrophie blanche, varicose veins, ankle flare and varicose eczema (*Figures 4.1–4.3*). The presence of these findings may suggest venous ulceration but does not confirm it. Neither does the site of ulceration, for although most venous ulcers will occur in the medial gaiter area they may also occur in any part of the lower limb including the foot (Morison and Moffatt, 1994) (*Figure 4.4*).

Venous ulcers were once thought to be relatively painless. This is now known not to be the case; up to 80% of patients with venous leg ulceration experience some discomfort and in 20% pain may be unremitting and severe (Franks *et al*, 1994). Noonan and Burge (1998) have recently confirmed this. It may, therefore, be impossible — on symptoms and signs alone — to distinguish between ulcer types.

Table 4.1: Factors that could give rise to complications

1 Patient's medical condition

i.	Arterial disease
ii.	Diabetes
iii.	Neuropathy
iv.	Cardiac failure
v.	Malignancy
vi.	Rheumatoid arthritis
vii.	Steroid therapy
viii.	Burns, scars and skin grafts

2 Leg shape

i.	Thin
ii.	Fat
iii.	Hourglass
iv.	Straight
v.	Oedematous

3 Patient's attitude

i.	Noncompliance
ii.	Uncomfortable
iii.	Socially unacceptable

4 Bandage

i.	Inappropriate bandage
ii.	Poor technique
iii.	Sensitivity to component

Vascular assessment

Routine assessment of the circulation of the lower limb should include palpation of ankle pulses and the observation of capillary perfusion, blanching, the presence of varicose veins and venous flares. This alone is, however, inadequate to define either the presence or absence of arterial or venous disease.

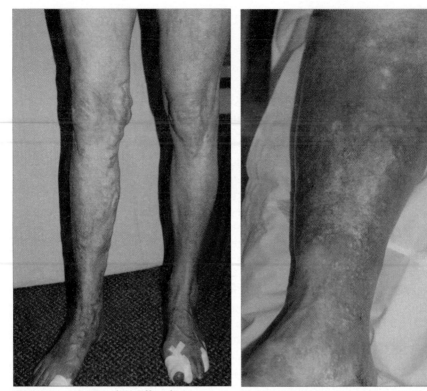

Figure 4.1: Gross clinically obvious varicose veins due to saphenofemoral incompetence

Figure 4.2: Extensive pigmentation associated with early lipodermato-sclerosis and atrophie blanche in a patient with gross deep and superficial venous reflux

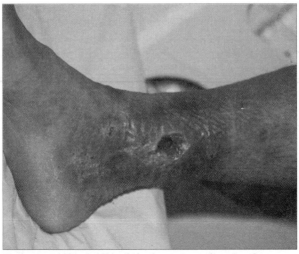

Figure 4.3: Typically placed venous ulcer in the medial gaiter area

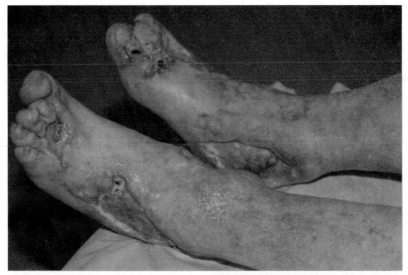

Figure 4.4: Bilateral long-standing chronic venous ulceration involving the foot and submalleolar areas

Doppler ultrasound

The use of the handheld Doppler provides an objective assessment of peripheral perfusion, though it is an unreliable method of assessing the extent of venous disease in the complex situation that may be encountered in a patient with a leg ulcer. When using the handheld Doppler to assess venous disease status the patient should stand. The leg to be examined should be relaxed and the knee slightly flexed. The patient's weight should be on the opposite leg. To test for reflux, place the probe over the common femoral or popliteal vein and manually compress and then release the calf muscles (*Figure 4.5*). Prolonged audible retrograde flow indicates reflux and the test can be repeated further down the venous system in an attempt to isolate the source of this reflux. If reflux is still detected when the superficial system has been occluded with a tourniquet it is likely to be within the deep system. By

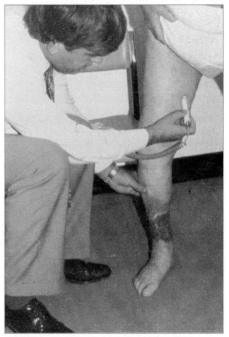

Figure 4.5: Using the hand-held Doppler to assess superficial venous reflux in the long saphenous vein

moving the tourniquet progressively down the leg it is possible to isolate sites of perforator incompetence but accurate localisation of perforating veins is often not possible with the continuous wave Doppler. It is frequently not possible to define accurately the site of reflux in the popliteal fossa, duplex colour flow ultrasonography being the investigation of choice in this situation.

The ankle brachial pressure index (ABPI)

Measurement of the ABPI is required in all patients before the application of compression bandaging. The method to be employed has been published by Vowden *et al* (1996) and is set out in *Box 4.2* and *Figures 4.6* and *4.7*. ABPI measurements should be used as part of the structured assessment of a patient with a leg ulcer.

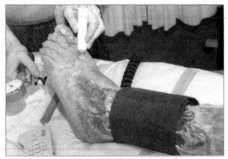

Figure 4.6: Position of the cuff and Doppler when recording the dorsalis pedis arterial pressure

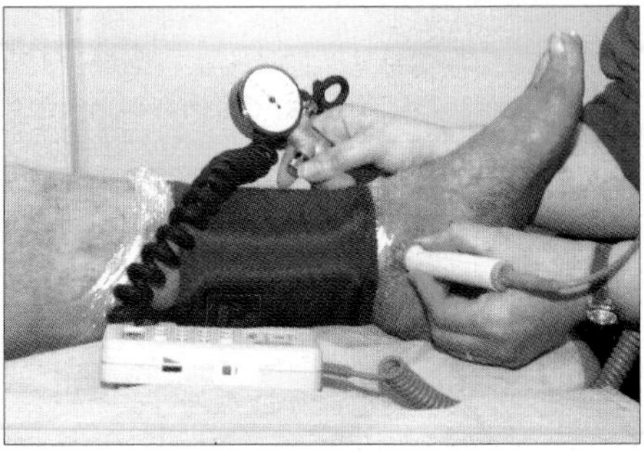

Figure 4.7: Position of the cuff and Doppler when recording the posterior tibial arterial pressure

Recommendations suggest that, as a general rule, an ABPI of 0.8 or greater will allow the safe application of high compression-bandaging (RCN Institute, 1998; SIGN, 1998). The potential problems associated with Doppler and ABPI calculations have been discussed in Vowden and Vowden (2001b).

Additional information on the state of the circulation can be derived from the signal analysis, the simplest form of which is operator interpretation of the audible signal (*Figure 4.8*) (Vowden, 1997; Faris *et al*, 1992). Alternatively, the waveform may be visualised and the Doppler spectrum analysed. This can be particularly useful in patients with non-compressible arteries, such as some patients with diabetes and renal failure. Alternative assessment methods include the use of the Pole test (Smith *et al*, 1994) and the measurement of toe pressures using either Doppler ultrasound, strain gauge plethysmography or laser Doppler (Vowden, 1999; Ramsey *et al*, 1988). The development of portable 'vascular laboratories' such as the Assist™ (Huntleigh Diagnostics) provides a means by which some of these more complex vascular investigations can be performed outside of a specialist unit.

Box 4.2: Doppler method

Explain the procedure and reassure the patient and ensure that he/she is lying flat and is comfortable, relaxed and rested with no pressure on the proximal vessels.

1. Measure the brachial blood pressure, as recommended by the British Hypertension Society:

    ❖ Place an appropriately sized cuff around the upper arm
    ❖ Locate the brachial pulse and apply ultrasound contact gel
    ❖ Angle the Doppler probe at 45° and move the probe to obtain the best signal
    ❖ Inflate the cuff until the signal is abolished then deflate the cuff slowly and record the pressure at which the signal returns being careful not to move the probe from the line of the artery

    Repeat the procedure for the other arm
    Use the **highest** of the two values to calculate the ABPI*

2. Measure the ankle systolic pressure:

    ❖ Place an appropriately sized cuff around the ankle immediately about the malleoli, for a normal sized ankle this will be a standard arm cuff, having first protected any ulcer that may be present
    ❖ Examine the foot, locating the dorsalis pedis (DP) and/or anterior tibial (AT) pulse and apply contact gel (*Figure 4.6*)
    ❖ Continue as for the brachial pressure, recording AT or DP pressure in the same way

    Repeat this for the posterior tibial (PT) (*Figure 4.7*) and if required the peroneal arteries
    Use the highest reading obtained to calculate the ABPI for that leg
    Repeat for the other leg
    Calculate the ABPI for each leg using the formula below or look up the ABPI using a reference chart
    For each leg, ABPI = highest ankle pressure (AT/PT/DP and/or Peroneal) for that leg
    Highest of the brachial systolic pressures for each arm

ABPI normally >1.0

ABPI <0.9 indicates some arterial disease

ABPI >0.5 and <0.9 can be associated with claudication and if symptoms warrant a patient should be referred for further assessment

ABPI <0.5 indicates severe arterial disease and may be associated with gangrene, ischaemic ulceration or rest pain and warrants urgent referral for a vascular opinion

Problems and errors may arise if:

1. The cuff is repeatedly inflated or inflated for long periods this can cause the ankle pressure to fall.

2. The cuff is not placed at the ankle. Ankle systolic pressure is not measured, pressure recorded is usually higher than ankle pressure.

3. The pulse is irregular or the cuff is deflated too rapidly. The true systolic pressure may be missed.

4. The vessels are calcified (diabetics), the legs are large, fatty or oedematous, the cuff size is too small, or the legs are dependent.
    Inappropriately high reading will be obtained.

*ABPI = ankle brachial pressure index

Duplex ultrasound

Duplex colour-flow ultrasound examination can provide both functional and anatomical information on the peripheral arterial and venous circulation. In real time the technique uses short pulses of ultrasound and can identify tissue boundaries, eg. vessel walls, blood flow, the duration and velocity of blood flow and reveal turbulence. Colour-flow duplex provides three types of information (*Figure 4.9*):

⌘ A B-mode or grey-scale image (a). Tissue interfaces reflect varying amounts of ultrasound. By plotting these on a brightness scale according to the quantity of reflected ultrasound a picture is assembled which gives anatomical detail.

⌘ A colour map is then overlayed on the anatomical detail (b, c). This is a representation of the Doppler frequency shift where velocity and direction of flow are allocated a colour from a preset colour scale.

⌘ Finally, Doppler spectral flow data (d) is obtained by 'sampling' from within the vessel of interest. This can be plotted against time to give information on flow velocity, direction and duration.

Venous ultrasound

Duplex ultrasound provides a convenient method by which to assess the venous system. Areas of valvular incompetence in both the superficial, junctional and deep veins can be identified along with thrombus, occlusion and recannulation. Using this technique it has been confirmed that almost 50% of all venous leg ulcers are a result of isolated superficial venous incompetence (Ghauri *et al*, 1996, 1998b). Recognition of the role of isolated superficial venous incompetence in ulcer disease allows surgical intervention which may reduce the incidence of ulcer recurrence (Ghauri *et al*, 1998b).

Arterial ultrasound

Using this same technique detailed information on the peripheral arteries can be obtained and areas of stenosis or occlusion identified. It has been established that this is an alternative to conventional arteriography in some patients (Guest *et al*, 1999b). This investigation can be useful in patients with suspected arterial disease in whom intervention by either angioplasty or bypass may be appropriate and has the advantage of being non-invasive. Alternative arterial imaging techniques include arteriography and magnetic resonance imaging (MR angiography). These are however costly and, in the case of arteriography, invasive.

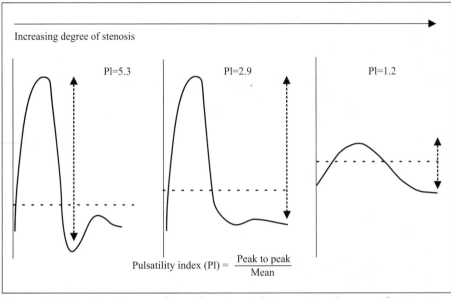

Figure 4.8: The Doppler waveform changes with increasing degrees of stenosis

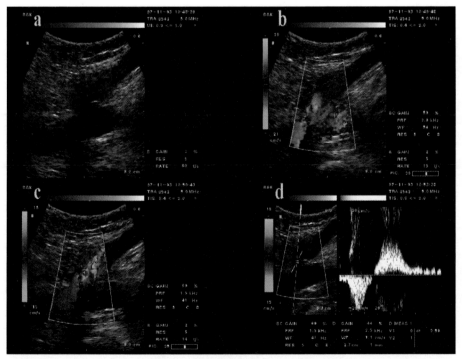

Figure 4.9: Colour flow duplex ultrasound of the saphenofemoral junction demonstrating and quantifying venous reflux

Other methods of venous assessment

Further information on the venous system may be needed in some patients and can be derived from a number of different modalities which include; venography, plethysmography, photoplethysmography, isotope studies, laser Doppler and venous pressure measurements. Venous pressure is measured by inserting a needle, connected to a pressure transducer and pen recorder, into a vein at the ankle or in the dorsum of the foot. The baseline pressure is recorded with the patient standing; the pressure is then recorded while the patient does ten toe-heel exercises, finally the recovery phase is recorded (Vowden, 1998). The resultant measurements reflect:

1. The efficiency of the calf muscle pump.
2. The degree of outflow resistance.
3. The presence or absence of reflux and its severity if present.

Photoplethysmography (PPG) and light reflective rheography (LRR) can be used non-invasively to assess refilling time. In both techniques a photodetector placed on the skin of the foot or ankle captures reflected infrared light. Increasing venous blood in the superficial skin vessels will alter the light transmission and reflection, so allowing venous refilling after exercise to be quantified. A typical result for a normal patient and one with significant reflux is shown in *Figure 4.10*. It has been suggested that this method of investigation could be used as a screening test for superficial and deep reflux and, as it is readily portable, it may provide a method for community-based screening (Moffatt *et al*, 2001).

Venography used to be more frequently performed, but its role has now largely been replaced by duplex ultrasonography and D-dimer assay for the detection of deep vein thrombosis (Bradley *et al*, 2000). Ascending venography remains a standard method for identifying and localising venous outflow obstruction, the most common cause of which is either an acute deep vein thrombosis or the consequence of an earlier thrombosis. Ascending venography is also useful to localise perforator incompetence and can provide the anatomical information necessary when complex venous reconstructive surgery is planned. Descending venography can provide additional anatomic information necessary for reconstructive surgery and will provide the functional information on valvular competence. Radionucleotide venography provides an alternative and reliable method of diagnosing major vein occlusion.

The interrelationship of the more commonly performed vascular investigations for the patient presenting with a leg ulcer is given in *Figure 4.11*.

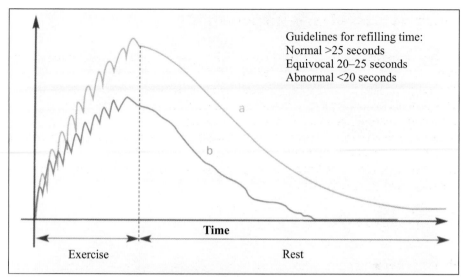

Guidelines for refilling time:
Normal >25 seconds
Equivocal 20–25 seconds
Abnormal <20 seconds

Figure 4.10: Venous reflux detected by photoplethysmography. Note the rapid refilling in the patient with venous valvular incompetence (b) compared to the normal subject (a) after ten heel-to-toe exercises

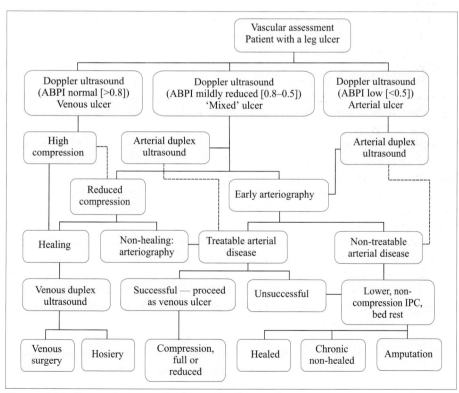

Figure 4.11: Suggested vascular investigation and management strategy for a patient with a presumed venous leg ulcer

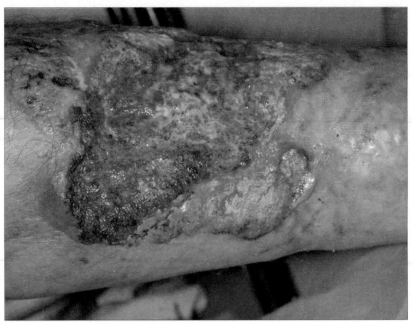

Figure 4.12: Malignant ulcer developing in an area of previously grafted venous ulceration. Only repeated biopsies revealed this to be a squamous cell carcinoma

Lower limb swelling

Limb swelling is a common finding in patients with lower limb ulceration. Patients with lymphoedema may require additional investigation of the lymphatic system to establish the cause of the limb swelling. This may include: limb volume measurement which can either be measured by displacement or by taking a series of circumference measurements which, in effect, treat the limb as a series of truncated cones; lymphangiography; lymphoscintigraphy; pelvic ultrasound and computerised tomography or magnetic resonance imaging (Mortimer, 1997).

Ulcer assessment

Tracings, particularly using a grid film, and simple linear measurements are frequently used to calculate ulcer area and describe ulcer size. However, scaled photography provides the best method of ulcer documentation and can allow analysis of ulcer bed for slough, assessment of the effectiveness of debridement and measurement of the rate of ulcer healing. For most ulcers this will be the only investigation of the ulcer itself that is required. Ulcers with an unusual appearance, ulcers not responding to treatment or ulcers in patients in whom a vasculitis is suspected should be biopsied, if need be repeatedly as small punch biopsies may miss an area of malignancy within a large ulcer (*Figure 4.12*). Malignancy has been reported to be present in 4.4% (Yang *et al*, 1996) and 6% of leg ulcers (Taylor *et al*, 1997). This worryingly high figure indicates the importance of reassessment in this group of patients with chronic wounds and the need for biopsy when ulcers do not behave in a predicted fashion.

The wider recognition of the importance of skin allergy and the development of hypo-allergenic products has reduced the incidence of allergic reactions to products. The skin surrounding the ulcer may, however, still cause concern and when this occurs patch testing may be appropriate (Cameron, 1998).

Swab

In the absence of overt signs of infection, such as cellulitis, pyrexia, increasing discharge, ulcer deterioration, increasing pain or odour, routine wound swabs are not required (Cutting and Harding, 1994; RCN Institute, 1998; Gilchrist, 1999). When these signs are present wound swabs should be taken in a structured manner following a defined protocol that has been agreed locally. The use of quantitative bacteriology has been suggested as a reliable way of defining wound infection and may be usefully combined with wound biopsy (Stotts, 1995). The methods involved, however, are costly and tend to be impractical.

Patient assessment

Blood pressure, weight and urinalysis should be taken routinely (RCN Institute, 1998). Specific haematological and biochemical investigations may be suggested by both the history and physical examination of the patient. These may include haemoglobin, urea and electrolytes, blood glucose and glycosylated haemoglobin (HbA1c) estimation. It may also be necessary to investigate the patient's nutritional status (Mulder *et al*, 1998) and his/her mobility as both are factors which can adversely affect wound healing. Patients with significant underlying medical conditions will also need specific assessment related to their underlying disease. This may include podiatric assessment of the diabetic foot including sensory testing, inflammatory marked measurement in patients with rheumatoid arthritis or other causes of a vasculitis, and cardiac investigations for patients with significant lower limb oedema and heart failure.

Conclusion

Investigations should be an aid to diagnosis and contribute to the correct management of the patient, the ulcer and the underlying disease process. For patients presenting with an uncomplicated venous ulcer the investigations necessary are measurement of the ankle systolic pressure and calculation of the ABPI, which should be repeated as part of a reassessment process; an assessment of the deep and superficial venous systems, ideally by colour-flow duplex ultra-sonography; and accurate documentation of the limb and ulcer. Complicated ulcers or venous ulcers that fail to respond to treatment will require more extensive investigation and assessment by specialist teams.

Key Points

❖ Assessment is at the heart of the classification and management of leg ulcers.

❖ A wide variety of techniques are available to permit correct diagnosis of the origin of an ulcer and the underlying disease process.

❖ No technique on its own is capable of identifying ulcer aetiology, and in the case of complex ulcers, several investigations may be necessary to reach a conclusion.

❖ Ongoing assessment is necessary to monitor the progress of any underlying vascular disease.

References

Baker SR, Stacey MC (1994) Epidemiology of chronic leg ulcers in Australia. *Aust NZ J Surg* **64**(4): 258–61

Bjellerup M (1997) Hydrostatic leg ulcers: a new classification. *J Wound Care* **6**(9): 408–410

Bradley M, Bladon J, Barker H (2000) D-dimer assay for deep vein thrombosis: its role with colour Doppler sonography. *Clin Radiol* **55**(7): 525–7

Browse NL, Burnand KG (1982) The cause of venous ulceration. *Lancet* **2**(8292): 243–5

Callam MJ, Ruckley CV, Dale JJ, Harper DR (1987) Hazards of compression treatment of the leg: an estimate from Scottish surgeons. *Br Med J Clin Res Ed* **295**(6610): 1382

Callam MJ, Ruckley CV, Harper DR, Dale JJ (1985) Chronic ulceration of the leg: extent of the problem and provision of care. *Br Med J* **290**(6485): 1855–6

Cameron J (1998) Skin care for patients with chronic leg ulcers. *J Wound Care* **7**(9): 459–62

Chant A (1990) Tissue pressure, posture, and venous ulceration. *Lancet* **336**(8722): 1050–1

Coleridge Smith PD, Thomas P, Scurr JH, Dormandy JA (1988) Causes of venous ulceration: a new hypothesis. *Br Med J* (Clin Res Ed) **296**(6638): 1726–7

Cornwall JV, Dore CJ, Lewis JD (1986) Leg ulcers: epidemiology and aetiology. *Br J Surg* **73**: 693–6

Cutting K, Harding KG (1994) Criteria for identifying wound infection. *J Wound Care* **3**(4): 198–201

Faris IB, McCollum P, Mantese V, Lusby R (1992) Investigation of the patient with atheroma. In: Bell PRF, Jamieson CW, Ruckley CV, eds. *The Surgical Management of Vascular Disease*. WB Saunders & Co, London

Franks PJ, Moffatt CJ, Connolly M *et al* (1994) Community leg ulcer clinics: Effect on quality of life. *Phlebol* **9**(2): 83–6

Ghauri AS, Grabs AJ, Nyamekye I, Poskitt KR (1996) Comparison of venous reflux in the affected and non-affected leg in patients with unilateral venous ulceration (letter; comment). *Br J Surg* **83**(9): 1305

Ghauri AS, Nyamekye I, Grabs AJ, Farndon JR, Poskitt KR (1998a) The diagnosis and management of mixed arterial/venous leg ulcers in community-based clinics (see comments). *Eur J Vasc Endovasc Surg* **16**(4): 350–5

Ghauri AS, Nyamekye I, Grabs AJ, Farndon JR, Whyman MR, Poskitt KR (1998b) Influence of a specialized leg ulcer service and venous surgery on the outcome of venous leg ulcers. *Eur J Vasc Endovasc Surg* **16**(3): 238–44

Gilchrist B (1999) Wound infection. In: Miller M, Glover D, eds. *Wound Management: Theory and Practice*. Nursing Times Books, London

Grabs AJ, Wakely MC, Nyamekye I, Ghauri AS, Poskitt KR (1996) Colour duplex ultra-sonography in the rational management of chronic venous leg ulcers. *Br J Surg* **83**(10): 1380–2

Guest M, Smith JJ, Sira MS, Madden P, Greenhalgh RM, Davies AH (1999a) Venous ulcer healing by four-layer compression-bandaging is not influenced by the pattern of venous incompetence. *Br J Surg* **86**(11): 1437–40

Guest M, Williams A, Greenhalgh R, Davies A (1999b) Mixed leg ulcers (letter; comment). *Eur J Vasc Endovasc Surg* **18**(6): 540–1

Higley HR, Ksander GA, Gerhardt CO, Falanga V (1995) Extravasation of macromolecules and possible trapping of transforming growth factor-beta in venous ulceration. *Br J Dermatol* **132**(1): 79–85

Lees TA, Lambert D (1992) Prevalence of lower limb ulceration in an urban health district. *Br J Surg* **79**(10): 1032–4

Moffatt C (1993) Assessing leg ulcers. *Pract Nurs* **21**: 8–10

Moffatt C (2001) Leg Ulcers. In: Murray S, ed. *Vascular Disease: Nursing and Management*. Whurr, London: 200–37

Moffatt CJ, Doherty DS, Franks PJ (2001) Non-invasive investigations of venous pathology in leg ulceration: A population study. (Abstract) Back to the Future 11th Conference of the European Wound Management Association, Dublin, Ireland

Morison M, Moffatt C (1994) *A Colour Guide to the Assessment and Management of Leg Ulcers*. 2nd edn. Wolfe Publishing, London

Mortimer P (1997) The swollen limb and lymphatic problems. In: Tibbs D, Sabiston D, Davies M, Mortimer P, Scurr J, eds. *Varicose Veins, Venous Disorders, and Lymphatic Problems in the Lower Limbs*. Oxford University Press, Oxford: 211–43

Mulder GD, Brazinski BA, Harding KG, Agren MS (1998) Factors influencing wound healing. In: Leaper DJ, Harding KG, eds. *Wound Biology and Management*. Oxford University Press, Oxford

Nelzen O, Bergqvist D, Lindhagen A (1994) Venous and non-venous leg ulcers: clinical history and appearance in a population study. *Br J Surg* **81**(2): 182–7

Noonan L, Burge SM (1998) Venous leg ulcers: Is pain a problem? *Phlebology* **13**(1): 14–19

Ramsey DE, Manke DA, Sumner DS (1988) Toe blood pressure. A valuable adjunct to ankle pressure measurement for assessing peripheral vascular disease. *J Cardiovasc Surg* **29**: 736

RCN Institute (1998) *Clinical Practice Guidelines: The Management of Patients with Venous Leg Ulcers*. RCN Institute, London

Salaman RA, Harding KG (1995) The aetiology and healing rates of chronic leg ulcers. *J Wound Care* **4**(7): 320–3

SIGN (1998) *The Care of Patients with Chronic Leg Ulcers*. SIGN Secretariat, Edinburgh

Smith FC, Shearman CP, Simms MH, Gwynn BR (1994) Falsely elevated ankle pressures in severe leg ischaemia: the pole test: an alternative approach. *Eur J Vasc Surg* **8**(4): 408–12

Stotts N (1995) Determination of bacterial burden in wounds. *Adv Wound Care* **8**(8): 46–52

Taylor A, Marcuson R, Whiteby C (1997) The importance of tissue biopsy for non-healing leg ulcers (abstract). In: Leaper D, Dealey C, Franks PJ, Hofman D, Moffatt CJ, eds. *New Approaches to the Management of Chronic Wounds*. Proceedings of the 7th European Conference on Advances in Wound Management. Macmillan, London

Vowden P (1997) Peripheral arterial disease. 2: anatomical investigations. *J Wound Care* **6**(3): 129–32

Vowden P (1998) The investigation of venous disease. *J Wound Care* **7**(3): 143–7

Vowden P (1999) Doppler ultrasound in the management of the diabetic foot. *Diabetic Foot* (1): 16–17

Vowden KR, Vowden P (1996) Peripheral arterial disease. *J Wound Care* **5**(1): 23–6

Vowden K, Vowden P (2001a) Mixed aetiology ulcers. *J Wound Care* **10**(1): 520

Vowden KR, Vowden P (2001b) Doppler and the ABPI: how good is our understanding? *J Wound Care* **10**(6): 197–202

Vowden KR, Goulding V, Vowden P (1996) Hand-held Doppler assessment for peripheral arterial disease. *J Wound Care* **5**(3): 125–8

Yang D, Morrison BD, Vandongen YK, Singh A, Stacey MC (1996) Malignancy in chronic leg ulcers. *Med J Aus* **164**: 718–20.

5

Developments in wound care for difficult to manage wounds

Kate Ballard, Helena Baxter

Research and development in wound healing has ensured that issues relating to chronic wound management remain high in the nursing agenda. Since the advent of modern wound dressings, which retain a moist wound healing environment, work has continued to progress into more advanced, interactive products which aim to alter the wound bed in order to promote a suitable environment for cell migration and growth. Rapid wound healing is advocated and necessary to reduce morbidity and mortality in patients with large chronic wounds and to reduce the financial and manpower implications of long-term wound care in the hospital or community setting. Vacuum-assisted closure, artificial skins, growth factors and larval therapy are discussed in order to give an overview of some of the emerging practices being adopted for difficult to manage wounds.

Since Winter demonstrated the benefits of a moist wound healing environment in 1962, modern wound dressings have largely superceded the traditional dry gauze dressings. Although the advent of dressings such as hydrocolloids, hydro-polymers, gels, foams and alginates has improved wound care and wound healing outcomes, there are still wounds which require rapid re-granulation to prevent further morbidity/mortality, and some which remain static and unresponsive to standard wound healing techniques.

Wound care is an ever-evolving field, and this chapter aims to explain some of the new technologies and fashions in wound care.

Vacuum-assisted closure

Vacuum-assisted closure (VAC; KCI Medical Ltd) is a relatively new concept designed to achieve rapid wound healing in acute and chronic wounds. The concept is simple — a uniform negative pressure is applied to the wound bed through an open cell porous foam which fills the cavity of the wound. A drainage tube is then inserted and the whole system is sealed, and kept in place, by a semi-permeable film dressing (*Figures 5.1* and *5.2*).

It is thought that the VAC system improves wound healing by removing excess exudate and stimulating angiogenesis (Morykwas *et al*, 1997) (*Figure 5.3*). Excess chronic wound fluid suppresses cell growth and proliferation. During early animal studies of the VAC system it was observed that there was a 63.3% increase in the rate of granulation tissue formation (Morykwas *et al*,

1997). Later, human studies in chronic wounds demonstrated that bacterial colonisation of the wound bed was reduced 1000 times after four days of treatment (Collier, 1997). The negative pressure system can reduce localised oedema resulting in increased blood flow at the wound bed, thereby increasing wound healing. This also increases the wound bed's resistance to infection by creating a hostile environment for bacterial growth.

VAC therapy has been shown to be effective in a variety of wounds, particularly surgical dehiscence, pressure sores, leg ulcers and diabetic foot ulcers (Baxandall, 1997; Collier, 1997). In the authors' experience, application of the VAC, both pre- and post-split skin grafting, has improved take-rates of the graft to 90–100%. It is, however, contraindicated in malignant wounds since it encourages

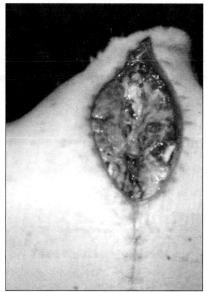

Figure 5.1: Wound before vacuum-assisted closure

growth of malignant cells as well as healthy cells, and it should be used with caution on patients with bleeding problems.

Although the cost of consumables for VAC therapy may appear to be high in relation to conventional dressings, in the authors' experience the whole therapy is cost-effective since it promotes rapid wound healing and the dressing can be left in place for two to four days. Patients generally find the system extremely comfortable and acceptable, and since the launch of the Mini-Vac™, the system is more portable and can facilitate early discharge from hospital.

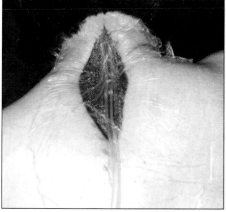

Figure 5.2: Vacuum-assisted closure *in situ*

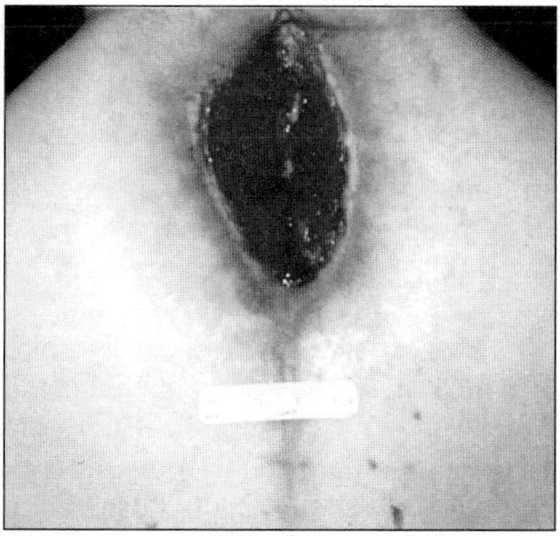

Figure 5.3: Healthy granulation bed following vacuum-assisted closure

Hyaluronic acid

Hyaluronic acid has been used successfully for many years in the field of opthalmology and in connective tissue diseases such as rheumatoid arthritis and inflamed joint conditions (Goa and Benfiled, 1994). It has also been used in the treatment of leg ulcers (Ortonne, 1996). Hyaluronic acid is a naturally occurring extra cellular matrix molecule and a major component of human skin. Recent research has been directed towards its role in

Table 5.1: Functions of hyaluronic acid in wound healing
Clot stabilisation
Maintenance of a moist wound environment
Facilitating cell proliferation and migration
Tissue hydration
Proteoglycan organisation in tissue repair
Improving the quality of tissue repair

Ballard and Baxter, 1999

wound healing, where it is thought to have the functions listed in *Table 5.1*.

Additionally, hyaluronic acid has been shown to enhance angiogenesis (West *et al*, 1985) and improve the phagocytic response of macrophages (Bernake and Marwald, 1979; Ahlgren and Jarstrand, 1984). It is a naturally occurring bio-degradable polysaccharide and is non-immunogenic. Therefore, an elephant's hyaluronic acid can be used for human wound healing with no immune response. The umbilical cord, synovial fluid, vitreous humor in the eye, and rooster combs are particularly rich in hyaluronic acid (Abatangelo *et al*, 1994).

ConvaTec has developed a new wound dressing (Hyalofill™), an absorbent fibrous fleece composed of an ester of hyaluronic acid. When Hyalofill is in contact with serum or wound exudate, a hydrophilic gel is produced which overlays the wound and creates a hylauronic acid rich tissue interface and moist wound environment conducive to granulation and healing. In appearance and management of exudate, it is much like a gel-forming alginate or hydrofibre.

The Hyalofill stimulates the wound and facilitates the development of a well vascularised dermal bed. In *Figure 5.4*, the patient had Hyalofill applied to just the upper portion of the recalcitrant arterial ulcer and the stimulation of the wound bed is clearly visible just 48 hours after application.

Hyalofill was originally used as a primer for two to three weeks before grafting with autologous keratinocytes (Vivoderm Autograft System; Beldon 1998). Research by Navsaria (1998) has shown that on full-thickness wounds, the 'take rates' of keratinocytes are significantly improved if the wound is pre-treated with Hyalofill.

Hyalofill has been used on various wound types (Ballard and Baxter, 1999). The most dramatic results have been noted in chronic, recalcitrant ulcer beds, wounds which are slow to heal and appear to be 'stuck' in the inflammatory stage of healing (Ballard and Cantor, 2002; Ballard and Baxter, 2000; Cantor, 2001a/b; Edmonds and Foster, 2000; Foster *et al*, 1999; Hollander *et al*, 2000a/b; de Leon *et al*, 2001). Hyalofill kick starts the wound and results are visible even after one dressing change. Hyalofill is easy to use, conforms well to the contours of the wound and can be cut to suit various wound shapes without shedding fibres or causing damage to surrounding skin.

Tissue engineering

Much finance and interest has recently been invested in tissue engineering and the development of 'manufactured skins'. Skin grafts have been used for many years in the realms of burns and plastic surgery. Autologous skin grafts usually involve taking large areas of the patient's own skin from a donor site, usually the back or thigh, to cover the area of deficit. For years, scientists have been trying to culture and grow keratinocytes in the laboratory (Rheinwald and Green, 1975) for autografting, and allografting, ie. replacing the patient's epidermal loss with genetically unrelated cells.

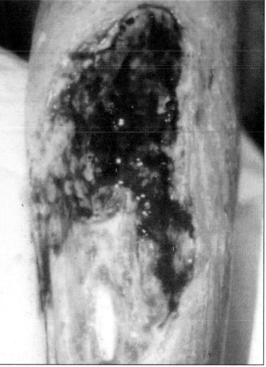

Figure 5.4: Hyalofill — revascularisation of arterial ulcer

A dermal replacement is more difficult to culture and recent clinical success has been through providing 'scaffolds' to aid the patient's own repair process. The following are examples of manufactured skin substitutes, and these are probably just the tip of the iceberg as research into this field progresses.

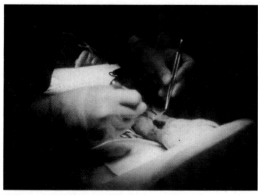

Figure 5.5: Cultured kertinocytes — Vivoderm graft application

Vivoderm Autograft System (Fidia Advanced Biopolymers) can be used to provide keratinocyte autografting for coverage of areas of skin loss without the need to create a donor site. The patient's own cells are cultured onto a hyaluronic acid scaffold for grafting (*Figure 5.5*). The cells are harvested from an 8mm skin biopsy and the keratinocytes are cultured and migrate through a laser-cut membrane. From a small biopsy, epithelial skin sufficient to cover an adult body can be generated in one month. The apparent advantage of Vivoderm autografting is that actively migrating and proliferating cells are delivered to the wound — potentially leading to a more efficient graft take and therefore wound closure. The take of the cultured keratinocytes on full-thickness wounds is, however, dependent upon a well vascularised, clean wound bed (Boyce and Holder, 1993).

Dermagraft™ (Smith & Nephew) is a living, bioengineered human dermal replacement. Dermagraft actually replaces the patient's damaged or destroyed dermal tissue with a healthy living human dermis which stimulates the patient's own epithelial cells. Human fibroblast cells are cultured from the foreskins of neonates onto a bioabsorbable scaffold of vicryl mesh. (A single donor foreskin provides sufficient cell seed to produce 250000 square feet of finished Dermagraft tissue; McColgan *et al*, 1998). As the fibroblasts proliferate onto this mesh, they secrete dermal collagen, growth factors and extracellular matrix proteins, creating a living dermis. The resulting metabolically active Dermagraft is then implanted into the chronic wound to facilitate healing. Dermagraft has been documented as being used successfully on long-standing neuropathic ulcers (Gentzkow *et al*, 1996).

Apligraf™ (Novatis) is an allogenic, bilayered tissue engineered skin that was developed for the treatment of chronic, difficult to heal ulcers. This tissue engineered skin consists of an epidermal layer formed of viable keratinocytes and a dermal layer composed of viable fibroblasts dispersed in a type I collagen matrix. Published work on Apligraf includes a large randomized controlled trial on venous leg ulcers, and on neuropathic diabetic foot ulcers (Falanga, 1998).

Tissue engineered skin can provide wound coverage especially in the cases of large burns where coverage is paramount to prevent dehydration and infection, and can create the microenvironment to stimulate healing. Integra™ artificial skin (Johnson & Johnson Medical) is a dermal template. It consists of two layers: a three-dimensional collagen dermal matrix; and a temporary silicone epidermal layer. It controls moisture loss from the wound and assists in closure of the wound bed by infiltration of the new dermis scaffold (Sheridan *et al*, 1994).

Identification of ulcers with a poor prognosis or those that have not adequately responded to conventional therapy can prompt the use of alternative, more appropriate advanced therapies, such as tissue engineered skin. These systems are expensive (£250–£1000 per graft) and are susceptible to destruction by colonising bacteria. However, these costs are offset by improving clinical outcomes and quality of life, resulting in a reduction in healthcare costs.

Larval therapy

Larval therapy (maggot therapy or biosurgery) is not a new concept in wound healing. Its use has been documented back to the First World War and the American Civil War, when it was noted that wounds infested (usually accidentally) with maggots were generally cleaner and had less infection than uninfested wounds (Thomas *et al*, 1998; Jones and Andrews, 1999).

The advent of the antibiotic era in the 1940s saw the decline of larval therapy as an adjunct to wound healing, but in the past five years it has enjoyed a fashionable comeback as a safe, non-surgical debriding agent with no known side-effects or allergies, with the added bonus of reducing bacterial count in wounds, including methicillin-resistant *Staphylococcus aureus* (MRSA) (Courtney, 1999).

Although accidental infestations of maggots still occur from time to time, planned interventions use sterile larvae of *Lucilia sericata* (greenbottle) from the Biosurgical Research Unit (BRU) in Bridgend. These larvae produce powerful enzymes which breakdown dead tissue and leave healthy granulation tissue unharmed (Jones and Andrews, 1999). It is also thought that these enzymes have the ability to combat clinical infection (Thomas *et al*, 1998) (*Figure 5.6*).

Successful use of larval therapy does, however, require some 'pet care' and the provision of a suitable environment. Hard, necrotic eschars are difficult for larvae to penetrate and may require some softening first. Any dressing materials left in the wound bed, such as hydrogels, may be detrimental to the larvae, and excessive exudate may cause them to drown (Vowden and Vowden, 1999). Conversely, without the provision of some moisture, the larvae will dry out and die. This is particularly relevant when considering the use of pressure-relieving equipment, since some therapies (eg. air-fluidised therapy) use warmed air which causes rapid dessication of the young larvae.

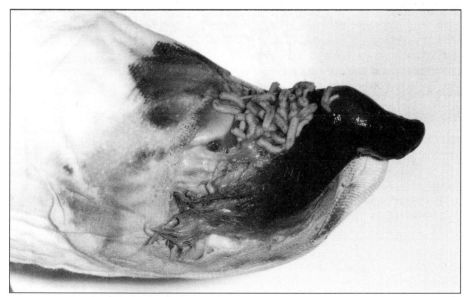

Figure 5.6: Larval therapy: maggots *in situ*

Sharp debridement may be considered to be the fastest method of removing dead/sloughy tissue, but is not always appropriate or without complications. Larval therapy offers a suitable and safe alternative, and can be used in all manner of wounds from pressure sores and leg ulcers to fungating lesions and osteomyelitis (Thomas *et al*, 1998; Jones and Andrews, 1999).

Growth factors

Much of the future treatment of chronic, recalcitrant wounds is in the development of topical products containing growth factors. There are many different growth factors involved in wound healing, such as platelet-derived growth factor (PDGF) which has been reported to promote angiogenesis, re-epithelialisation and granulation tissue formation (Hart, 1999), epidermal growth factor (EGF), primarily involved in accelerated epidermal regeneration (Cox, 1993), and transforming growth factor (TGF-B) which may be involved in many wound healing processes, and has been shown to enhance healing even when the normal healing processes are impaired (Cox, 1993).

The use of topical growth factors in chronic wounds is based on the assumption that many wounds require a trigger to stimulate the normal healing process (Graham, 1998). This has been shown to be both statistically and clinically significant in a study using a PDGF gel in chronic neuropathic diabetic ulcers (Wieman *et al*, 1998). This multi-centre, randomised, double-blind study showed improved rates of wound closure and a decrease in the time taken to achieve wound closure when using a PDGF-based gel compared to a placebo gel.

At present, topical growth factors are being used in clinical practice more as an 'experimental' approach to problematic wounds. There is still only a small body of evidence from phase III and IV trials available to support the use of the various growth factors in the healing of chronic wounds. Further research is needed before the use of growth factors is likely to be widely adopted (Hart, 1999). One question in need of clarification is which growth factor is required at which stage of wound healing, since some growth factors can be inhibitory or stimulating depending upon the local wound environment (Graham, 1998).

One reason why growth factors may not work in chronic ulcers is that there are high levels of matrix metalloproteinases (MMPs), which break down growth factors and may contribute to the chronicity of some wounds. A new product called Promogran (J&J) is a MMP inhibitor and is currently being tried in clinical practice.

The future

The treatment of wounds has come a long way in the past thirty years, and is likely to continue to progress rapidly with advancing technology and greater understanding of chronic wound states. Nursing focus should, however, retain the basics of good wound care (nutrition, hygiene, mobility, psychological support and education). The future for patients with large or chronic wounds is getting brighter, with faster wound healing, reduction in morbidity and mortality, restoration of function and improved cosmetic results.

Early indications of future developments include dipsticks for wound growth factors to identify stages of healing, spray skins which produce a collagen scaffold, and anti-scarring agents for the prevention and treatment of hypertrophic and keloid scars. Advances in genetic research may produce gene transfer techniques (introduction of DNA or RNA molecules into cells), which could inhibit or stimulate specific cellular functions. This may have great potential for the treatment of wounds with biochemical or genetic defects.

As these 'tomorrow's world' therapies and treatments evolve, they will hopefully be accompanied by the futuristic techniques to cure the underlying wound aetiologies — as prevention is always better than cure in these chronic debilitating wounds that have such an impact on a patient's quality of life.

Key points

❖ Some wounds remain static and unresponsive to standard wound healing techniques.

❖ Wound care is an ever-evolving field.

❖ Larval therapy is re-emerging as a successful therapy.

❖ Artificial skin substitutes and growth factors are being manufactured for use on acute and chronic wounds.

❖ Vacuum-assisted closure is a cost-effective method of encouraging healing in chronic wounds.

References

Abatangelo G, Brun P, Cortivo R (1994) Hyaluron (hyaluronic acid): an overview. Proceedings of workshop at Annual Meeting of the European Society for Biomaterials, Pisa, September, sponsored by ConvaTec

Ahlgren T, Jarstrand C (1984) Hyaluronic acid enhanced phagocytosis of human monocytes in vitro. *J Clin Immunol* **4**(3): 246–9

Ballard K, Baxter H (1999) A novel wound dressing. *Nursing Telegraft* (Burns and Plastic Surgery Nurses; BAPSN) 2(Spring/Summer): 5–7

Ballard K, Baxter H (2000) Developments in wound care for difficult to manage wounds. *Br J Nurs* **9**(7): 405–12

Ballard K, Cantor A (2002) A novel development in utilising hyaluronic acid. Hyalofill: an ester of hyaluronic acid for the treatment of recalcitrant diabetic wounds. *Ostomy Wound Manag*: in press

Baxandall T (1997) Healing cavity wounds with negative pressure. *Elderly Care* **9**(1): 20–2

Beldon P (1998) Management of a patient with a chronic venous ulcer using a new autologous skin graft system. European Wound Management Association (EUMA) 8th European Conference on Advances in Wound Care, Harrogate, 17–19 November

Bernake DN, Marwald RR (1979) Effects of hyaluronic acid on cardiac cushion in collagen matrix cultures. *Texas Respiratory Biological Medicine* **39**: 271–85

Boyce ST, Holder IA (1993) Selection of topical antimicrobial agents for cultured skin for burns: combined assessment of cellular cytotoxicity and antimicrobial activity. *Plast Reconstr Surg* **92**(3): 493–500

Cantor AJ (2001a) Management of a five-year-old venous ulcer with a hyaluronic acid based dressing in an immunocompromised patient: a case history. Poster presentation, Symposium for Advanced Wound Care, Las Vegas, April 2001

Cantor AJ (2001b) Preventing amputation by using proper wound care: a case history. Poster presentation, Symposium for Advanced Wound Care, Las Vegas, April 2001

Collier M (1997) Know how: Vacuum-assisted closure (VAC). *Nurs Times* **93**(5): 32–3

Courtney M (1999) The use of larval therapy in wound management in the UK. *J Wound Care* **8**(4): 177–9

Cox D (1993) Growth factors in wound healing. *J Wound Care* **6**: 339–42

De Leon JM, Lucius A, Fudge PT, Brister K (2001) Hyaluronic acid dressing (Hyalofill) in a complex wound of the hand: a case history. Poster presentation, Symposium for Advanced Wound Care, Las Vegas, April 2001

Edmonds M, Foster A (2000) Hyalofill: a new product for chronic wound management. *Diabetic Foot* **3**(1): 29–30

Falanga V (1998) Apligraf treatment of venous ulcers and other chronic wounds. *J Dermatol* **25**: 812–17

Foster AM, Bates M, Doxford M, Edmonds ME (1999) The treatment of indolent neuropathic ulceration of the diabetic foot with Hyaff. *Diabet Med* **16**: S94

Gentzkow G, Iwasaki S, Hershon K *et al* (1996) Use of Dermagraft: a cultured human dermis to treat diabetic foot ulcers. *Diabetes Care* **19**: 350–4

Goa KL, Benfiled P (1994) Hyaluronic acid: a review of its pharmacology and use as a surgical aid in opthalmology and its therapeutic potential in joint disease and wound healing. *Drugs* **47**: 536–66

Graham A (1998) The use of growth factors in clinical practice. *J Wound Care* **7**(9): 464–6

Hart J (1999) Growth factors. In: Miller M, Glover D, eds. *Wound Management*. Nursing Times Books, London: 153–69

Hollander DA, Schmandra T, Windolf J (2000a) A new approach to the treatment of recalcitrant wounds: a case report demonstrating the use of a hyaluronan ester fleece. *Wounds* **12**(5): 111–7

Hollander DA, Schmandra T, Windolf J (2000b) Using an esterified hyaluronan fleece to promote healing in difficult-to-treat wounds. *J Wound Care* **9**(10): 463–6

Jones M, Andrews A (1999) Larval therapy. In: Miller M, Glover D, eds. *Wound Management*. Nursing Times Books, London: 129–33

McColgan M, Foster A, Edmonds M (1998) Dermagraft in the treatment of diabetic foot ulcers. *The Diabetic Foot* **1**(2): 75–8

Morykwas M, Argenta L, Shelton-Brown E *et al* (1997) Vacuum-assisted closure: a new method for wound control and treatment: animal studies and basic foundation. *Ann Plastic Surg* **38**(6): 553–62

Navsaria HA (1998) An *in-vitro* study to demonstrate pre-treatment of full-thickness wounds with Hyalofill significantly improves the take rates of cultures keratinocytes in porcine model. Oral presentation, British Burns Association 31st Annual Meeting, 15–17 April

Ortonne JP (1996) A controlled study of the activity of hyaluronic acid in the treatment of venous leg ulcers. *J Dermatol Treatment* **7**: 75–81

Rheinwald JG, Green H (1975) Formation of a keratinizing epithelium culture by a cloned cell line derived from a teratoma. *Cell* **6**: 317–30

Sheehan C, Meneses P, Ennis WJ (2001) Hyaluronnan in the management of recalcitrant venous ulcers. Poster presentation, Symposium for Advanced Wound Care, Las Vegas, April 2001

Sheridan RL, Hegarty M, Tompkins RG, Burke JF (1994) Artificial skin in massive burns results to ten years. *Eur J Plast Surg* **17**: 91–3

Thomas S, Andrews A, Jones M (1998) The use of larval therapy in wound management. *J Wound Care* **7**(10): 521–4

Vowden K, Vowden P (1999) Wound debridement 1: non-sharp techniques. *J Wound Care* **8**(5): 237–40

West DC, Hampson LN, Arnold F *et al* (1985) Angiogenesis induced by degradation products of hyaluronic acid. *Science* **228**: 1324

Wieman TJ, Smiell J, Su Y (1998) Efficacy and safety of a topical gel formulation of recombinant human platelet-derived growth factor-BB (Becalpermin) in patients with chronic neuropathic diabetic ulcers. *Diabetes Care* **21**(5): 822–7

Winter G (1962) Formulation of the scab and the rate of epithelialization in the skin of the domestic pig. *Nature* **193**: 293–4

Section III:
Acute wounds

6

Acute surgical wound care 1: an overview of treatment

Peter Moore, Lorraine Foster

This chapter traces the history of surgical wound care, from primitive dressings and techniques of closure used in the past to the present-day approach. The history of surgical wounds is discussed together with a classification of the different types of surgical wound closure. Nowadays, it is recognised that the management of surgical wounds has to be planned carefully to achieve adequate exposure to the area of surgery. At the same time the surgeon has to be conscious of how the wound will heal to ensure optimal postoperative function and cosmetic results. To do this an understanding of the principles underpinning surgical incisions, and of alternative techniques for their closure, drainage and wound dressing, is needed. The role of the nurse in preparing patients preoperatively and supporting and caring for them postoperatively is paramount.

Most surgical wounds are the result of a planned procedure, either elective or emergency, where the surgeon creates the wound in order to perform a surgical procedure. However, wounds may also be caused by trauma, such as a road traffic accident, or a knife or gun-shot injury; in these cases the wound is already present when the surgeon sees the patient for the first time.

The latter type of wound requires a different approach from that used for a planned incision. Factors such as the site of the wound, the presence or absence of infection, and the possibility of contamination by dirt or clothing need to be considered when managing these wounds, as they have not been created under the sterile conditions of the operating theatre.

Prehistoric and primitive healing

Surgery is as old as man itself, and is estimated to date from around half a million years ago, from the time when Java man (*pithecanthropus erectus*) evolved (Haeger, 1988). Early surgery was probably devoted to tending wounds. Little is known of how it was practised during prehistoric times. It is likely, however, to have been performed in more or less the same way as it is carried out by primitive folk today. It is common for most primitive tribes to cover wounds with leaves and other parts of plants to effect healing.

Filling wounds with spider webs was a popular method of treatment. This is an instinctive process, which is not based on evidence but on custom and

practice passed on from generation to generation. Shakespeare refers to this in
A Midsummer Night's Dream:

> *I shall desire of you more acquaintance good master cobweb.*
> *If I cut my finger I shall make bold of you.*
> *A Midsummer Night's Dream*, III. i

Indeed, little boxes containing spider webs were part of every soldier's
equipment at the battle of Crécy in 1346, and we still use dressings with a
web-like pattern to dress wounds and absorb exudate today.

Our ancient ancestors also realised the value of draining the wound. The
letting of pus that has collected is an old surgical custom. The Dakota Indians
sharpened a feather quill and mounted it on an animal bladder. The quill was
stuck into the afflicted area and the pus sucked up into the bladder, allowing a
free outlet for fluid and pus. The same principle is followed today, the difference
being that we now use sterile tubes and drainage bags.

Early man was also aware of the benefit of closing large wounds. In the
past, Masai tribes in Africa put a large Acacia thorn through both edges of the
wounds and then pulled the ends together using twine plant fibres — the
equivalent of our modern-day sutures.

Yet the prize for inventiveness must surely be awarded to the tribes of India
and South America, where the surgeon brought the wound edges together and his
aide allowed a termite or beetle to bite across them. When the insect had taken a
good bite his neck was twisted quickly. The jaws stiffened in death and made a
perfect wound clamp! This principle is still in use today when metallic clips are
applied to skin wounds (Haeger, 1988).

Surgical wounds today

Moy (1993) defines acute wounds as:

> *A destruction in the integrity of the skin including the epidermis and
> dermis.*

He goes on to state that:

> *Healing is the reparative process by the skin to protect itself and deeper
> structures.*

Surgical and nursing interventions in wound care can greatly affect the result of
the scar and the time to healing. This chapter will discuss wounds seen on an
acute general surgical ward. Other types of wounds, such as burns, which require
specialised reconstructive skills and nursing support under the care of plastic
surgeons, and certain chronic wounds (eg. leg ulcers and bedsores) encountered by
dermatologists, vascular surgeons and community physicians and nurses, which
present specialised problems, are not discussed here.

Planning the wound

When a surgeon is performing an operation, consideration needs to be given to various aspects of the incision (*Table 6.1*).

Exposure

The object of the incision is to allow adequate exposure to the area of surgery so that the correct procedure can be performed safely. In the past, surgical folklore stated that surgeons should be

Table 6.1: Factors associated with the planning of acute surgical wounds
Exposure
Postoperative function
Pain
Cosmesis

generous in their incision, because wounds healed from side to side, not from end to end (Lord, 1971, personal communication). This resulted in the surgical aphorism 'big mistakes are made in little holes'.

More recently, nurses and surgeons have realised that although wounds heal from side to side, 'they hurt from end to end' (Lord, 1971, personal communication). This has led to surgical operations being carried out through smaller incisions, ie. laparoscopic (keyhole) surgery, which allows procedures to be completed through tiny incisions with less disruption and pain in the postoperative period (*Figure 6.1*).

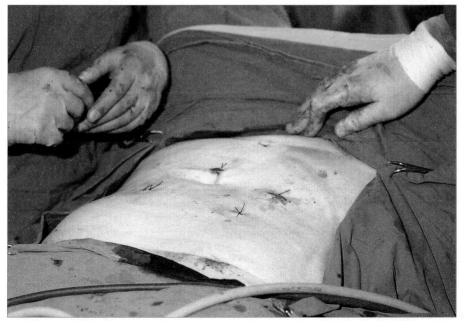

Figure 6.1: Laparoscopic surgery

Postoperative function

Although the surgeon is primarily concerned with gaining access to the tissues when making the incision, consideration also has to be given to how the wound will heal. This primarily concerns function following surgery. For example, incisions made at right angles across joints tend to contract with healing, thus restricting the range of movement of the joint postoperatively (Fisk, 1979).

Pain

Patients should not experience pain postoperatively. A report from the Joint Commission of the Royal College of Surgeons and College of Anaesthetists in 1990 stated that postoperative pain was generally inadequately recognised, recorded, monitored or treated (Royal College of Surgeons of England, 1998).

The situation has since improved with advanced technology, such as the use of patient-controlled analgesia (PCA) (Alexander, 1993). Research has shown that patients receiving PCA experience pain relief most of the time (Thomas, 1993). This is supported by nurses, who believe that PCA gives patients control of their pain and reduces their anxiety (Thomas, 1993).

It is vitally important to control pain postoperatively, as pain can decrease oxygen uptake, increase mortality and morbidity, increase susceptibility to tumour progression, and delay mobility, increasing the length of hospital stay (Alexander, 1993).

Certain incisions are notoriously painful, eg. a vertical abdominal incision hurts more than a transverse abdominal incision. The reason for this is that a vertical incision transects more nerve endings than a transverse incision, as pain nerves run circumferentially around the body from the spinal cord (Ellis, 1974).

Postoperative pain relief may therefore be achieved not just by analgesia and reassurance from the medical and nursing staff on the ward, but also by judicious planning of the wound in the operating theatre (Wall and Melzack, 1995). Freedom from pain enables the patient to mobilise freely and recuperate quicker, thus reducing the risk of postoperative complications such as chest infection, deep vein thrombosis and pulmonary embolism (Ellis and Calne, 1977).

Cosmesis

The appearance of the scar is important. Wounds that are made along natural contours, ie. Langer's lines (Gibson, 1978), heal better with a neater scar than incisions that cross Langer's lines. The best way to work out the direction of these lines is to look at the direction of hair growth on the skin. In general, the hairs on the skin grow along Langer's lines, providing a guide to the most cosmetic incision (Burnand and Young, 1992).

Both doctors and nurses must bear in mind that the scar of surgery is permanent and that patients will only have to look at their scar to remind them of their experiences.

Principles of closing surgical wounds

Once the surgical procedure has been completed the surgeon must decide what to do with the open wound. Usually the wound is closed and the skin brought together; this is known as healing by first or primary intention (Dealey, 1994) (*Figure 6.2*). The aim is to bring the deep tissues and then the skin together in anatomical layers without tension. This is usually achieved by suturing, with obliteration of the dead space (the gap between the tissues). Finally the skin is closed. A variety of methods are available for this purpose, eg. sutures and clips.

Sometimes it is not possible to obliterate all the dead space and there is a possibility of build-up of bodily fluid, eg. blood, serum or pus. In this case, the surgeon will consider the use of a drain to enable the accumulated fluid to drain away, allowing the deeper tissues to heal.

A drain may also be inserted as a safety measure in the event of problems with surgery performed in the deeper tissues. For example, a drain may be inserted near a bowel anastomosis, which would probably heal uneventfully. However, if breakdown and leakage of bowel contents were to occur, the drain would allow these to drain externally. Thus, the catastrophic effects of leakage and spillage of intestinal contents within the abdomen, which would result in peritonitis, a lethal condition, would be avoided.

Some wounds cannot be closed safely, and the surgeon therefore elects to leave them open to allow them to heal naturally (Foster and Moore, 1997). This is known as healing by secondary intention (*Figures 6.3* and *6.4*), and is commonly used for infected or contaminated wounds (Marks *et al*, 1985).

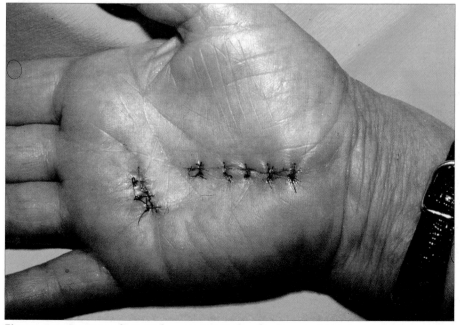

Figure 6.2: A sutured wound — an example of primary closure

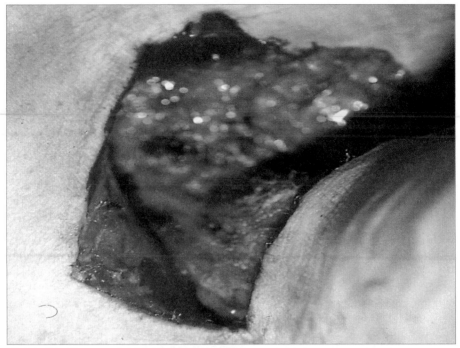

Figure 6.3: Open wound — infected axilla

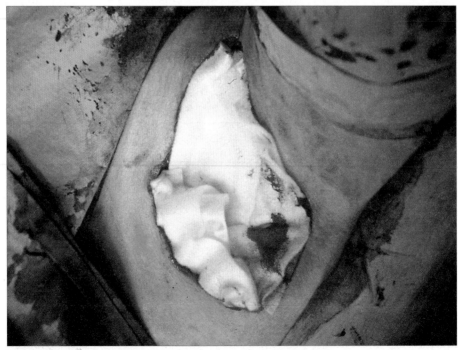

Figure 6.4: Open wound with a hydrofibre dressing in place

An example of an infected wound would be an open wound following drainage of a superficial abscess, eg. ischio-rectal abscess or pilonidal sinus. An example of a contaminated wound would be a penetrating wound resulting from trauma, which might contain soiled clothing. The surgeon would expect these wounds to be dirty and infected, and would therefore perform the operation with the intention of leaving them open because further infection and build-up of pus would be anticipated. Under these circumstances, if the wound was closed then a further abscess might develop, necessitating a second procedure to drain the pus. Leaving the wound open allows free drainage.

Sometimes an interoperative problem may occur which prevents the wound from being closed. For example, if uncontrollable bleeding is encountered during surgery the surgeon may have no choice but to pack the wound tightly to arrest haemorrhage, and leave this pack in position at the end of the surgical procedure. In such cases the wound is left open so that the pack can be retrieved at a later date when the blood vessels have sealed off and haemorrhage is no longer a problem.

In wounds that are left open, the choice of dressing and the nursing care are very important (Moore and Foster, 1997). In surgical wounds that are left open to heal by secondary intention the surgeon does have an alternative choice, ie. to consider closing the wound by suture at a second surgical procedure when the infection, contamination or bleeding has settled. This is known as delayed primary closure. The different types of wound closure are listed in *Table 6.2*.

Table 6.2: Types of healing of acute surgical wounds
Primary — close approximation of the wound edges and deep structures
Primary closure with drainage of deep cavities
Healing by secondary intention, especially infected/contaminated wounds
Delayed primary closure when contamination is cleared

Certain surgical procedures are carried out in several stages. An example of this is reconstructive surgery following operative surgery for malignant disease, eg. breast reconstruction following mastectomy. In this case, the reconstructive surgeon will not only have to consider the type of wound closure to use, but also will be using devices that will expand the tissue. The purpose of this is to expose a new tissue plain for insertion of a prosthesis, muscle tissue, etc. in order to restore body contours that have been destroyed by the original surgery for cancer.

Conclusion

The creation of a surgical wound and its subsequent healing require a great deal of thought for optimum results. In this chapter, we have discussed aspects of surgical techniques, 741 planning, and the creation and closure of acute surgical wounds.

The role of the nurse extends way beyond this. From the preoperative period, she/he will be preparing the patient for surgery, giving care and advice on such issues as pain management, tissue viability and nutrition. Postoperatively, advice will be given on care and the management of wound dressings throughout the recovery period.

Physical and psychological support will also be needed to ensure optimum wound healing. This may involve specific nursing roles such as stoma care and other clinical nurse specialist skills. These require specialist training, which is outside the scope of this chapter (Foster *et al*, 1997; Kaur, 1997).

Key points

❖ Modern acute surgical wounds are defined and compared and contrasted with the historical approach.

❖ The role of the surgeon and the position of the surgical wound are important in planning the surgical incision.

❖ When closing surgical wounds the surgeon must decide whether to close the wound by primary closure, or primary closure with drainage.

❖ Alternatively, healing by secondary intention or delayed primary closure may be the preferred option.

References

Alexander JI (1993) Postop pain control. In: Taylor I, Johnson CD, eds. *Recent Advances in Surgery*. Churchill Livingstone, London: 1–16

Burnand KG, Young AE (1992) *The New Aird's Companion in Surgical Studies*. Churchill Livingstone, London

Dealey C (1994) *The Care of Wounds: A Guide for Nurses*. Blackwell Scientific Publications, Oxford

Ellis H (1974) *Clinical Anatomy*. Blackwell Scientific Publications, Oxford: 58–60

Ellis H, Calne R (1977) *Lecture Notes in General Surgery*. Blackwell Scientific Publications, Oxford: 18–28

Fisk GR (1979) *Operative Surgery (Orthopaedics Part 2)*. Rob C, Smith R, eds. Butterworths, London: 525–6

Foster L, Moore P (1997) The application of a cellulose based dressing in the management of acute surgical wounds. *J Wound Care* **6**(10): 469–73

Foster L, Flood A, Moore PJ (1997) The evolving role of the surgical nurse practitioner in the acute setting In: Sanderson D, Brown J, eds. Managing Medicine: A Survival Guide. *Financial Times*, London: 93–102

Gibson T (1978) Karl Langer and his lines. *Br J Plast Surg* **31**(1): 1–2

Haeger K (1988) *The Illustrated History of Surgery*. Nordbok, Gothenberg, Sweden: 9–33

Kaur S (1997) The evolving role of the nurse practitioner in endoscopy. In: Sanderson D, Brown J, eds. Managing Medicine: A Survival Guide. *Financial Times*, London: 103–14

Marks J, Harding KG, Ribeiro CD (1985) Pilonidal sinus excision — healing by open granulation. *Br J Surg* **72**: 637–40

Moore P, Foster L (1997) The use of a modern hydrofibre dressing in surgical wounds. Oral presentation at the 7th European Conference on Advances in Wound Management, Milan

Moy LS (1993) Management of acute wounds. *Wound Healing* **11**(4): 759–60

Royal College of Surgeons of England (1990) *Commission on the Provision of Surgical Services: Report of the Working Party on Pain after Surgery*. Royal College of Surgeons, London

Thomas N (1993) Patient and staff perceptions of PCA. *Nurs Standard* **7**(28): 37–9

Wall PD, Melzack R (1995) *Textbook of Pain*. Churchill Livingstone, London: 377–8

7

Acute surgical wound care 2: the wound healing process

Peter Moore, Lorraine Foster

The previous chapter on acute surgical wound care traced the history of surgical wound care from primitive dressings and techniques of closure used in the past to the present-day approaches. It also outlined the classification of acute surgical wounds. This chapter describes the four stages of wound healing in acute surgical wounds, using clinical slides to illustrate the wound healing process. General factors, such as age, nutrition and medication, and local factors, including a moist environment, blood supply and wound infection, will be discussed to demonstrate their importance in promoting optimum wound healing.

In order to improve their skills in assessment and decision making with regard to wound care, nurses need to have a thorough understanding of how wounds heal. There is clear evidence that, although nurses are knowledgeable about the wound healing process, they often fail to apply this knowledge in practice (Lomas, 1988). By improving their knowledge, nurses may be able to reduce the amount of time spent on wound care, ensuring more effective use of resources and reducing the length of hospital stay for patients while promoting a pain-free recovery (Foster *et al*, 1998).

Wound healing

For optimum wound healing there has to be a balance of nutrition, tissue oxygenation and removal of debris in an occlusive environment (Chang *et al*, 1996).

Wound healing can be viewed as taking place in four overlapping stages (Davidson, 1992; *Table 7.1*). It occurs as the result of a complex interaction of cells.

Table 7.1: The four stages of wound healing
Haemostasis and inflammation
Granulation
Epithelialisation
Remodelling

Stage 1: haemostasis and inflammation

This first stage is the initial reaction to a surgical injury. *Figure 7.1* shows the open surgical wound following radical surgery. (Note the redness of the wound, and the darker areas where diathermy has been applied to cauterise the bleeding points.) The injured blood vessels release fibrinogen, which is converted to fibrin; this then forms a clot, resulting in haemostasis. At the same time, platelets release other chemical substances, including growth factors.

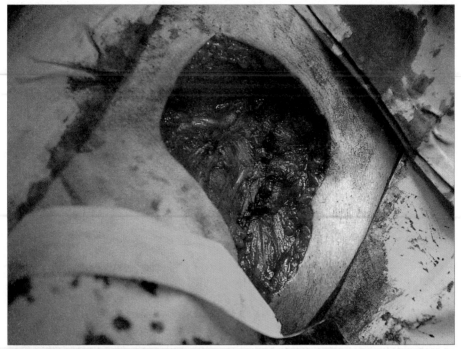

Figure 7.1: Open wound showing redness and bleeding points, demonstrating the need for haemostasis

These growth factors cause the severed blood vessels to constrict, thus stopping bleeding, and local blood vessels to dilate and become more porous. Dilatation of the local blood vessels causes a rise in the local temperature, leading to an increase in blood flow and erythema; pores between the endothelial cells enlarge and some of the contents leak into the surrounding tissues (extravasation). Oedema then ensues as a result of the vasodilatation and extravasation. Oedematous tissue press on the local nerve endings, causing pain. This sequence of events produces the clinical picture of inflammation. Loss of function is also a characteristic of this stage (Underwood, 1996).

Within hours of the wounding taking place, circulating polymorphonuclear neutrophils are attracted to this combination of chemical reactions and adhere to the endothelium of adjacent vessels. The polymorphonuclear neutrophils then migrate into the surrounding tissue to defend the body against microbial invasion by killing the micro-organisms and by phagocytosing debris.

This triggers the beginning of the second stage of healing — granulation. The polymorphonuclear neutrophils and the macrophages both release enzymes to destroy the micro-organisms and phagocytose debris. In turn, the macrophages and activated platelets begin to secrete a combination of growth factors which initiates the healing process.

Stage 2: granulation

In this stage of the healing process, growth factors and other intercellular signalling molecules from macrophages, endothelial cells and platelets attract dermal fibroblasts. This process in turn stimulates growth factors and synthesis of collagen matrix, through which new blood vessels will develop. All these elements will then form granulation tissue, until it is covered with a new epithelium.

The above process takes one to four days (Keen, 1981). New capillary loops will form, giving a red granular appearance to the new dermis. The wound edges may be drawn inwards owing to a signalling of mediators which organise their actin and myosin bundles into contractile organs; this is particularly noticeable in full-thickness wounds. At this point the wound is contracting and starting to look smaller. *Figure 7.2* shows the appearance of a wound at three days; note that the wound edges are starting to draw inwards.

Stage 3: epithelialisation

Once the new dermis approaches the level of the original skin, nature then uses another method of wound closure, termed epithelialisation. The combination of the growth factor cocktail from the inflammatory macrophages and fibroblasts and the new dermis, which is rich in collagen, hyaluronan and fibronectin, causes hair follicles, sebaceous glands and sweat glands to migrate over the dermal surface and spread until the dermis is completely covered with a new epidermis.

Daughter cells are then pushed upwards away from the dermis where they lose their nuclei and flatten, forming the outer barrier known as the stratum corneum, which is clinically recognised as healed skin.

In total this process of epithelialisation takes between five and twenty days (Keen, 1981). The stratum corneum protects the body from external contaminants and provides an effective barrier to fluids. *Figure 7.3* illustrates the close proximity of the wound edges in a healed wound showing epithelialisation.

Stage 4: remodelling

This remodelling or maturation stage is the fourth and final stage of the healing process. It begins at approximately twenty-one days and can take from a couple of months to one year to complete.

After epithelialisation, granulation tissue is gradually replaced by a new collagen-containing extracellular matrix. The granulation tissue, which has been acting as the provisional dermis and is initially very fragile, may regain 80% of its original strength as the scar matures. There is some loss of elasticity, and in some circumstances this can cause adhesions or excessive contractures.

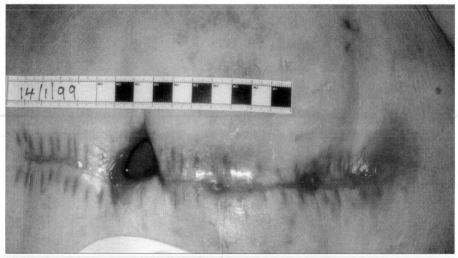

Figure 7.2: Cavity wound at three days showing granulation

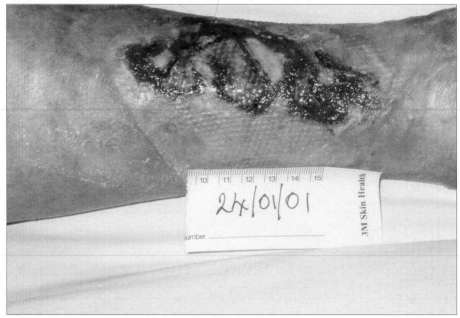

Figure 7.3: Cavity wound at three weeks showing epithelialisation

Other factors in wound healing

Other factors that influence wound healing can be divided into two groups: general factors and local factors (*Table 7.2*).

General factors

Age: In healthy young people the wound healing environment is ideal. The term 'healthy' does not simply refer to the patient's physical well-being, but includes social, psychological and emotional state.

The capacity of the wound to heal swiftly is dependent upon the age of the patient, as the skin loses its elasticity and becomes thinner with increasing age (Dealey, 1994).

General nutrition: Nutrition is very important in wound healing. A mal-

Table 7.2: Other factors to consider in wound healing	
General factors	Age
	General nutrition
	Medication
	Psychological state
Local factors	Site of the wound
	Moist wound healing
	Blood supply
	Wound infection
	Wound temperature

nourished state may provide inadequate amounts of protein for optimal wound healing. This leads to a decreased rate of collagen synthesis, resulting in a lower wound tensile strength and may increase the chances of wound infection (LaVan and Hunt, 1990).

Oxygen is essential for good wound healing. Consequently, tobacco smoke and nicotine, both of which cause vasoconstriction, resulting in a decrease in wound tissue perfusion, should be avoided (Silverstein, 1992).

Medication: Anti-inflammatory drugs, anticoagulants and glucocorticoids (steroids) are the drug classes that most commonly affect wound healing. Moy (1993) points out that steroids in particular reduce the inflammatory response, impair collagen synthesis and reduce resistance to infection.

Other immunosuppressive agents, such as those used in postoperative transplant surgery and cancer chemotherapy, also delay wound healing (Falcone and Nappi, 1984).

Psychological state: Recent studies support the theory that stress can inhibit the growth of fibroblasts, leading to delay in wound healing (Saito *et al*, 1997). Nursing care should focus on ensuring that patients are stress free, through good communication with patients and their carers.

Excessive pain can also cause local vasoconstriction and lengthen healing time. The nurse must ensure that patients' pain is kept under control at all times.

Local factors

Site of the wound: In general, wounds on the head and neck heal better than those in other areas, one reason being increased vascularity (Moy, 1993).

As explained in *Chapter 6*, the appearance of the scar is very important and wounds made along Langer's lines, which follow the natural contours of the body, heal with a neater scar.

Moist wound healing: Around the time of Hippocrates, it was documented that to prevent infection a wound had to be kept as dry as possible. The possibility that a moist environment might be important was first raised in 1948 when Gilge discovered that venous leg ulcers healed faster under Unna's boot if they were covered with moisture-retentive tape (Gilge, 1949).

This idea, however, was not accepted until 1962, when Winter applied this principle to swine wounds (Winter, 1962), signifying a breakthrough in the understanding of how wounds healed.

This work has been replicated on many occasions, on both deep and shallow wounds (Field and Kerstein, 1994), with good results. It is now accepted that in moist wounds the epithelial cells migrate more quickly, as they burrow beneath the underlying dermis (Thomas, 1990). *Figure 7.4* shows a cavity wound dressed with a modern dressing which keeps the wound moist and warm, providing optimal conditions for wound healing.

It is important to create a moist wound healing environment through the use of occlusive dressings or dressings that allow tissue hydration (Eaglestein, 1985). Eaglestein found that the use of an appropriate occlusive dressing accelerated wound healing by 40%.

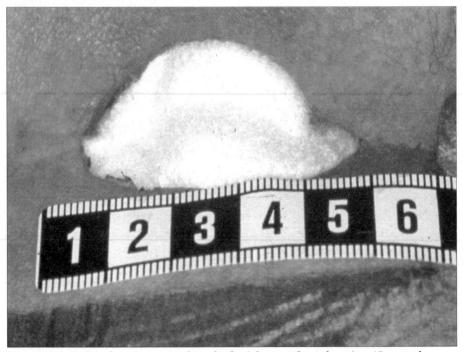

Figure 7.4: Surgical cavity wound packed with a modern dressing (Aquacel hydrofibre). Reproduced by kind permission of Dr JE Akerlund, Huddinge Hospital, Sweden

Blood supply: Ischaemic wounds heal more slowly than well-perfused wounds. Patients with local ischaemia, eg. those with peripheral vascular disease, are more prone to infection and frequent breakdown of surgical wounds (Forrest *et al*, 1981). However, even patients with well-perfused tissue may develop ischaemia when subjected to crude surgical technique involving crushing or dragging of the tissue during surgery.

Infection: All wounds are contaminated with a variety of micro-organisms, but most wounds do not become infected, although compromised vascularity can lead to invasion by pathogenic organisms.

Some clinicians have expressed concern about the effect of moisture-retentive dressings on wound infection. Ensuring that the wound is moist and warm would seem to favour the growth of pathogenic bacteria, leading to infection, but studies have shown this not to be the case (Hutchinson and Lawrence, 1991). Moy (1993) defines an infection as 'bacterial densities of more than 10000 organisms per gram of tissue'. In the presence of infection, wound healing is slowed due to the secretion of proteases by the infecting organisms, which injure the surrounding tissue, resulting in inflammation. Full infection with abscess formation and 10000 or more bacteria per gram of tissue requires antibiotics and drainage for wound healing.

Wound temperature: Research has shown that mitotic activity slows when the wound temperature is reduced (Myers, 1982). Lock (1980) found that after the wound had been redressed it took forty minutes for the wound temperature to return to normal and three hours for mitotic activity to return to normal.

Thus, for optimal wound healing it is essential to use the correct type of dressing to enable wound temperature to stay constant.

Summary

Wound management is the responsibility of the multidisciplinary team although the majority of the management is in the hands of the nursing profession. This chapter has given a brief overview of the wound healing process and some of the factors that should be considered when nursing patients with acute surgical wounds.

Key points

❖ The four main stages in wound healing are: haemostasis and inflammation; granulation; epithelialisation; and remodelling.

❖ General factors that must be considered when optimising the environment for wound healing include: age of the patient; nutritional status; concurrent medication; and the patient's psychological state.

❖ Local factors that should also be taken into account include: the site of the wound; local blood supply; wound infection; and wound temperature.

References

Chang H, Wind S, Morris D (1996) Dermatology nursing. *Moist Wound Healing* **8**(3): 174–6

Davidson JM (1992) Wound repair. In: Gallin JL, Goldstein LM, Snyderman R, eds. *Inflammation: Basic Principles and Clinical Correlates*. 2nd edn. Raven Press, New York: 809–19

Dealey C (1994) *The Care of Wounds*. Blackwell Scientific, London: 83–126

Eaglestein WH (1985) Experiences with biosynthetic dressings. *J Am Acad Dermatol* **12**: 434–40

Field C, Kerstein M (1994) Overview of wound healing in a moist environment. *Am J Surg* **167**(1a) Suppl: 2s–6s

Forrest APM, Carter DC, Macleod IB (1981) *Principles and Practice of Surgery*. 2nd edn. Churchill Livingstone, London: 131–42

Falcone RE, Nappi JF (1984) Chemotherapy and wound healing. *Surg Clin North Am* **64**: 779–94

Foster L, Moore P, Clark S (1998) The quality and cost benefits of the correct choice of dressing in the management of acute surgical wounds left to heal by secondary intention. Oral presentation, 8th European Conference on Advances in Wound Management, Madrid

Gilge O (1949) Ulcus cruris in venous circulatory disturbances. *Acta Derm Venereol* (Suppl) (Stockh) **29**(22): 13–28

Hutchinson JJ, Lawrence JC (1991) Wound infection under occlusive dressings. *J Hosp Infect* **17**: 83–94

Keen G (1981) *Operative Surgery and Management*. Wright PSG, London: 9–13

LaVan FB, Hunt TK (1990) Oxygen and wound healing. *Clin Plast Surg* **17**: 443–69

Lock PM (1980) The effects of temperature on mitotic activity at the edge of experimental wounds. In: Lundgren A, Soner AB, eds. *Symposia on Wound Healing: Plastic Surgical and Dermatological Aspects*. Molndal, Sweden

Lomas C (1988) Wound care supplement. *Nurs Times* **84**(38): 63–6

Moy SL (1993) Wound healing. *Manage Acute Wounds* **11**(4): 759–60

Myers JA (1982) Modern plastic surgical dressings. *Health Soc Serv J* **92**: 336–7

Saito T, Tazawa K, Yokoyarna Y, Saito M (1997) Surgical stress inhibits the growth of fibroblasts through the elevation of plasma catecholamine and cortisol concentrations. *Surg Today* **27**(7): 627–31

Silverstein P (1992) Smoking and wound healing. *Am J Med* **93**: 22–4

Thomas ST (1990) *Wound Management and Dressings*. Pharmaceutical Press, London

Underwood JCE (1996) *General and Systematic Pathology*. 2nd edn. Churchill Livingstone, London: 221

Winter GD (1962) Formation of a scab and the epithelialization of superficial wounds in the skin of the young domestic pig. *Nature* **193**: 293–4

8

Wound care in the accident and emergency department

Trudie Young

Wound assessment in the accident and emergency (A&E) department has a different focus from that in other clinical areas because of the lack of available clinical information about the patient. A wound may have had a greater physical impact than is immediately apparent and therefore a comprehensive skin assessment is often necessary. The wound will require thorough exploration and debridement to enable healing to take place with minimal complications. The methods of debridement and cleansing used in the A&E department are often unique because of the complexity of wound contamination. The variety of wounds encountered in this setting necessitate a large repertoire of dressing regimens. Modern wound management products can be adapted to meet the needs of the wounded patient in the A&E department.

Wound assessment requires a more enquiring approach in the accident and emergency (A&E) department than in other hospital departments. All patients attending a ward or outpatient clinic present with a past medical history and a reason for attendance. However, in the A&E department the patient's medical history is often unknown and the nurse does not have access to information that will indicate the cause of the patient's wound. This may be compounded by the patient's inability to provide a comprehensive history as a result of fear, anxiety, pain or alteration in neurological status. The nurse therefore has little information from which to work. This highlights the importance of an holistic patient assessment which incorporates a top-to-toe examination of the patient's skin status. The three main facts that need to be established are:

1. Where did the injury take place?
2. How did it happen?
3. When did it take place?

The answers to these questions will alert the nurse to the potential wound complications. The environment in which the injury occurred will indicate possible contamination and the foreign bodies that may be present in the wound. How it happened will indicate the patient's role and, as a consequence, his/her attitude to the wound. When it happened will identify the time lapse between the patient sustaining the injury and presenting in the department. The older the wound, the greater the risk of infection (Young, 1995). Although collection of data is important, it may have to take second place to primary patient assessment and physiological resuscitation. The wound history will therefore probably be collected during the second phase of the assessment.

Wounds assessed in the A&E department fall into four broad categories:

1. Non accidental injuries.
2. Superficial traumatic wounds.
3. Extensive traumatic wounds.
4. Covert traumatic wounds.

Wound assessment in A&E

Wound assessment in the A&E department differs from the assessment of routine postoperative or chronic wounds. The wound induced by trauma may have hidden depths and cannot be treated in isolation: its underlying or adjacent tissues must also be assessed. The first part of the assessment establishes the amount of tissue loss and, if possible, the damage to the other tissue. Once this information has been established, the clinician will then be in a position to limit further tissue injury to the initial wound (Wijetunge, 1992).

Detailed examination of the wound may require the use of a local or general anaesthetic. Once the wound area is anaesthetised exploration of the wound can begin. Any damage to deep structures must be identified and the viability of all tissue types in the area established, eg. muscle and tendon. Prior to administration of an anaesthetic agent the neurological status of the tissue adjacent to the wound should be tested for altered sensory perception.

The results need to be analysed carefully. In hand injuries, sensation may be present for a few hours after injury, even in the presence of digital nerve damage. In certain situations, eg. puncture wounds, exploration can cause more damage, and in these situations the necessity for wound exploration has to be justified (McCreadie, 1993). X-rays can be utilised to demonstrate the presence of radiopaque foreign bodies, but will not detect radiolucent items such as wood, thorns and splinters.

Debridement

Following assessment the second stage of wound care is debridement. It is essential that, where possible, all foreign bodies, contaminating substances and devitalised tissue are removed. The process of debridement can range from a simple hand wash to more complex surgical debridement under general anaesthetic.

Whiteside and Moorehead (1994a) classify wounds as tidy or untidy. A tidy wound has a clean incision, uncontaminated, caused by low energy trauma and presents to the A&E department within six hours of its occurrence. An untidy wound has a ragged edge, is contaminated, caused by high energy trauma, and presents to the A&E department more than twelve hours after its occurrence.

The degree of wound debridement is directly related to the category of wounds: tidy wounds can be cleansed by irrigation with warm/tepid water or saline, whereas untidy wounds will require more extensive cleansing and debridement. Cleansing the wound may start with cleaning the surrounding skin, especially if it is covered with oil or grease. Petroleum distillates are frequently selected as the solutions of choice for removal of grease. However, these solutions should not come into contact with the wound bed. In animal models a positive correlation has been established between the use of petroleum distillates and adverse tissue reactions (Thompson *et al*, 1990).

Certain types of debris can be removed by manually scrubbing the wound bed. This technique does, however, cause a local increase in tissue oedema (Whiteside and Moorehead, 1994b) and hydrogen peroxide provides a suitable alternative. When hydrogen peroxide solution comes into contact with the wound bed, oxygen bubbles are liberated rapidly and this acts as a mechanical detergent, lifting the debris from the wound bed. Due to the risk of embolus formation, hydrogen peroxide must be used with care when applied under pressure in closed cavities (Thomas, 1990).

The cleansing process should not be tissue toxic or increase wound inflammation, as this results in a decreased ability to deal with the bacteria in the wound bed (Chisholm, 1992). High pressure irrigation is advocated as an alternative method of dislodging debris from the wound bed. The optimum pressure can be achieved by using a 30ml syringe equipped with a 18–20 gauge needle. The syringe plunger should be depressed, using maximum force, at a distance of 2cm above the level of intact skin. If debris is not removed from the wound the cosmetic result will be poor, and the patient will be left with tiny, black, mottled marks. This is termed 'tattooing'.

Irrigation can be hazardous for the clinician by producing a splatter/splashback response. These hazards can be minimised by wearing eye protection throughout the procedure and replacing the needle with a quill. Alternatively, a commercially prepared spray cannister which delivers a saline jet at 6.88 psi at 37°C can be used (Williams, 1996).

The issue of maintaining asepsis throughout the cleansing procedure is questionable. To attempt asepsis before the majority of contaminating debris is removed is of negligible value. The sterility of the cleansing solution has also been brought into question following a study by Angeras *et al* (1992). In this study the authors compared the effectiveness of tepid water and sterile saline in the cleansing of soft tissue injuries in an A&E department. They found no increase in the infection rate in the wounds cleansed with tepid water. The use of tepid water also brings some normality into the cleansing process and, where possible, allows the patient to become involved in the process. This involvement may reduce patient fear and pain associated with the procedure.

Antiseptic solutions can be used as cleansing agents, but need to be in contact with the wound bed for an extended period to exert any benefit. These solutions are deactivated in the presence of organic matter such as blood (*Figure 8.1*) and pus which negates their value.

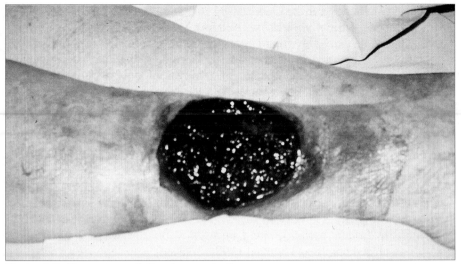

Figure 8.1: Haematoma following contusion

Wound management

Once cleansed, the wound will require a management strategy in order to promote healing, obtain an acceptable cosmetic result and enable the patient/affected area to return to full function.

Abrasions

These are sheering and friction injuries that result in a scraping or rubbing away of the epidermis or dermis (Flynn, 1994). These superficial wounds can be extremely painful owing to the presence of exposed nerve endings. An occlusive dressing, such as a hydrocolloid, is the dressing of choice for this type of wound. These dressings can be left in place for several days and the patient is able to bathe and shower with the dressing *in situ*. Traditionally, a non-adherent dressing was used for abrasions. When this dressing was compared with an extra-thin, hydrocolloid dressing in ninety-six patients with lacerations, abrasions or minor operative incision wounds, similar healing rates were obtained (Heffernan and Martin, 1994). However, those patients who used the hydrocolloid dressing showed a statistically significant reduction in their level of pain and in the amount of analgesia they required.

Paraffin tulle is also used for dressing traumatic excoriation. When it was compared with hydrocolloid dressings the latter were found to be less painful to remove (Andersson *et al*, 1991). The main problem identified by one patient who had sustained soft tissue injuries to the shoulder, neck and ear in a road traffic accident was the pain which resulted from the removal of paraffin gauze (Benbow, 1994). The location of these injuries rendered them unsuitable for the use of a hydrocolloid or film dressing. However, the injuries healed painlessly following the use of a hydrogel as the primary dressing. If the wound is on the patient's hand then a polyurethane membrane dressing will offer more limb flexibility than other dressings, thus lessening the risk of contractures (Williams, 1994).

Lacerations

These are open wounds with irregular tissue damage caused by sharp or dull objects in conjunction with tearing or shearing forces (Flynn, 1994). The aim of wound management is to reunite the opposing wound edges. However, this is not always possible and delayed closure may be necessary if there is a risk of infection (Berk, 1993). Wounds with the greatest potential for infection include those subject to gross contamination at the time of injury, bites, lacerations caused by a crush injury, and wounds that are presented more than six hours after the injury is sustained.

If wound closure is appropriate, then sutures, tissue adhesive or strips may be used, each method having advantages and disadvantages. Sutures are suitable for wounds that will be exposed to tension and movements, eg. over joints. Suturing is the preferred method of wound closure for facial wounds involving the lip, eyebrow and nostril because accuracy is vital in order to ensure a good cosmetic result. Sutures to a scalp wound can be reinforced by the use of hair knots.

Paper strips are suitable for small wounds with easily opposed edges, but are not suitable for wounds exposed to flexion (Cockerill and Sweet, 1993). They are particularly helpful in the closure of skin flap lacerations. Space should be left between strips to allow the drainage of exudate. The strips should not be covered by a film/hydrocolloid dressing as these may exacerbate the wound tear on removal (Krasner, 1991).

Tissue adhesives can be used for closing small wounds with tidy edges. Gulliver (1991) conducted a questionnaire survey of forty-two A&E departments in an attempt to establish a consensus on the use of tissue adhesives. However, responses to the questionnaire were diverse and often conflicting, and a consensus opinion was therefore unattainable.

Applebaum *et al* (1993) assessed the efficacy, comfort, cost-effectiveness and complications of tissue adhesives when used in the treatment of traumatic lacerations. They concluded that the technique was painless, with low complication rates, and was cost-effective because of the reduced need for follow-up visits, suture removal and anaesthesia. The patients indicated a high level of satisfaction with this method of wound closure. Tissue adhesive is more commonly employed in paediatric than adult settings and is mainly used for the treatment of small lacerations, especially those involving the face (excluding the eyelids and mouth).

A wound contact layer, eg. mepitel can be used as a primary wound dressing and covered by absorbent dressings. This is especially useful if the patient experiences pain on dressing removal, the wound contact layer will not adhere to the wound and dressing changes are pain free.

Avulsion injuries

These injuries are caused by shearing and tension forces that result in the tearing of tissue and full-thickness tissue loss (Flynn, 1994). The degloving injury is an extreme form of this type of wound. The amount of tissue loss usually necessitates wound healing by secondary intention, followed by skin grafting to achieve skin closure. Price and Thomas (1994) describe the use of a hydrogel to debride devitalised tissue in preparation for skin grafting.

Digit injuries

These injuries are more common than degloving injuries and involve a smaller amount of tissue loss, but are extremely difficult to dress. A thin hydrocolloid dressing or wound contact layer covered by low adherent dressing are easy to apply to this type of injury.

Puncture wounds

These are small external openings in the skin which damage and penetrate the underlying tissue (Flynn, 1994). Bites are a common cause of this type of wound. They require exploration to ensure that no fragments of tooth remain in the wound. Cat bites tend to cause deep punctures. If the area bitten involves the hand, there is the risk of tenosynovitis, septic joints and osteomyelitis (Anderson, 1992). Alginate dressings can be packed loosely into puncture wounds to facilitate removal of exudate. Magnesium sulphate paste was mythically reported to draw foreign bodies out of wounds (Leaman, 1991). On the whole bites are left to heal by secondary intervention. Cosmesis and restoration of function are two reasons for suturing of bite wounds. Antibiotic therapy is not necessary for all individuals. Higgins *et al* (1997) suggest it may be more cost effective to treat established infections rather than giving prophylactic antibiotic therapy to all recipients of bite wounds.

Crush injuries

These injuries are caused by a blunt object striking soft tissue over a bony surface (*Figure 8.2*). They may not initially present with a break in the skin surface, although the patient may sustain a wound if complications develop.

A serious complication associated with this type of wound is compartment syndrome. In this condition, pressure builds up within a limited space, ie. in the tissues, and compromises the circulation in this area. Although there is an increase in local blood flow it is insufficient to meet the increased metabolic needs of the muscle and nerves. The patient complains of severe pain disproportionate to the injury, pain on passive extension, local hyposthenia and muscle weakness. The emergency measure undertaken to relieve this complication is fasciotomy (*Figure 8.3*), which will eventually require skin grafting (Connolly, 1988).

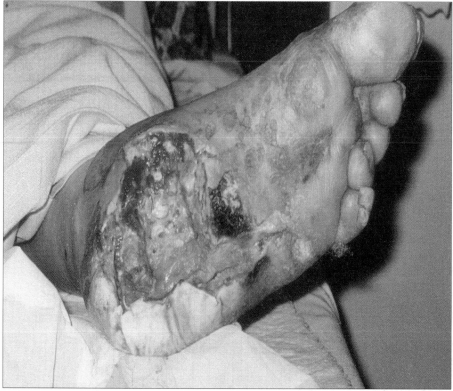

Figure 8.2: Crush injury

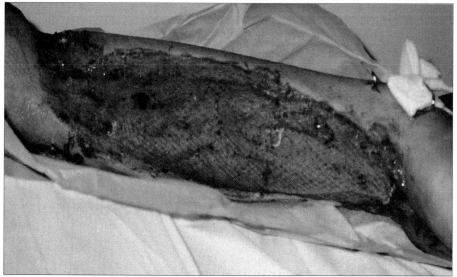

Figure 8.3: Fasciotomy after grafting

Conclusion

Wound management in the A&E department requires different wound assessment skills from those utilised when caring for a patient with a postoperative or chronic wound. The assessment in A&E is holistic and involves a top-to-toe examination of the patient's skin. Scarring and loss of limbs can result from inappropriate wound management. The clinician in the A&E department does not have the benefit of hindsight as he/she only sees the patient on one or two occasions and so the opportunity to evaluate wound care products is limited.

It is important that the A&E clinician knows which dressings are available for prescription by the GP if the patient is to receive subsequent wound management in the community. This information is available from the *Drug Tariff*.

Infection is one of the main complications of traumatic wounds and universal precautions must be stringently adhered to for the protection of all concerned.

Modern wound management products have a role to play in the healing of all types of traumatic wounds (Eyre, 1993; Young, 1995). The cost of newer products may affect their introduction into a clinical area, especially one that is renowned for its use of cheaper and more traditional products, eg. paraffin gauze. It is at this interface between quality of care and financial cost that responsibilities of staff become blurred and, if ignored, can lead to the patient becoming the victim.

Health promotion is a key aspect of A&E nursing and is important in the holistic management of traumatic wounds. Nurse-led minor injury clinics may be the appropriate place for this proactive approach to develop (Cable, 1995).

Traumatic wounds belong to traumatised patients and the skill of caring for them involves integrating the art of nursing and the science of wound healing.

Key points

❖ Thorough assessment and debridement of traumatic wounds is essential.

❖ Wound assessment may have to take second place to physiological resuscitation.

❖ Modern wound management products can be used in a variety of traumatic wounds.

❖ Scarring and loss of limbs can result from inappropriate wound management.

References

Anderson CR (1992) Animal bites. *Postgrad Med* **92**(1): 134–49

Andersson AP, Puntervold T, Warburg FE (1991) Treatment of excoriations with a transparent hydrocolloid dressing: a prospective study. *Injury* **22**(5): 429–30

Angeras MHA, Brandberg A, Falk *et al* (1992) Comparison between sterile saline and tepid water for the cleansing of acute traumatic soft tissue wounds. *Eur J Surg* **158**: 347–50

Applebaum JS, Zalut T, Applebaum D (1993) The use of tissue adhesion for traumatic laceration repair in the emergency department. *Ann Emerg Med* **22**(7): 1190–2

Benbow M (1994) Collaborative care of a patient with soft tissue injuries. *J Wound Care* **3**(2): 79–80

Berk WA (1993) Demystifying treatment of simple lacerations. *Emerg Med* **25**(2): 26–39

Cable S (1995) Minor injuries clinics: dealing with trauma. *Br J Nurs* **4**(20): 1177–82

Chisholm CD (1992) Wound evaluation and cleansing. *Emerg Med Clin North Am* **10**(4): 665–72

Cockerill J, Sweet A (1993) Nursing requirements of common accident wounds. *Br J Nurs* **2**(11): 578–82

Connolly JF (1988) Managing cuts and bruises. *Emerg Med* **20**(19): 78–100

Eyre G (1993) Alternative wound dressings in accident and emergency. *Nurs Standard* **7**(19): 25–8

Flynn MB (1994) Wound management of the traumatically injured patient. *Crit Care Nurs Clin North Am* **6**(3): 491–9

Gulliver G (1991) Sticking together. *Nurs Times* **87**(23): 74–8

Heffernan A, Martin AJ (1994) A comparison of a modified form of Granuflex (Granuflex Extra Thin) and a conventional dressing in the management of lacerations, abrasions and minor operation wounds in an accident and emergency department. *J Accid Emerg Med* **11**: 227–30

Higgins MAG, Evans RC, Evans R (1997) Managing animal bite wounds. *J Wound Care* **6**(8): 377–80

Krasner D (1991) An approach to treating skin tears. *Ostomy Wound Manage* **32**: 56–8

Leaman AM (1991) Wound care in the accident and emergency department. *Hosp Update* **17**: 422–8

McCreadie D (1993) Penetrating wounds. *Practitioner* **237**: 867–9

Price AS, Thomas S (1994) Care of the patient after a degloving of the leg injury. *J Wound Care* **3**(3): 129–30

Thomas S (1990) *Wound Management and Dressings*. The Pharmaceutical Press, London

Thompson W, Herschman B, Unthank P, Pieper D, Hawtof D (1990) Toxicity of cleansing agents for removal of grease from wounds. *Ann Plast Surg* **24**(1): 40–4

Whiteside M, Moorehead J (1994a) Traumatic wounds: care and management. *J Tissue Viabil* **4**(2): 48–50

Whiteside M, Moorehead J (1994b) Traumatic wound management. *J Wound Care* **3**(4): 183–6

Wijetunge D (1992) An accident and emergency approach. *Nurs Times* **88**(46): 70–6

Williams C (1994) Spyrosorb and Spyroflex. *Br J Nurs* **3**(12): 628–30

Williams C (1996) Irriclens: a sterile wound cleanser in an aerosol can. *Br J Nurs* **5**(16): 1008–10

Young T (1995) Traumatic wounds. *Pract Nurs* **6**(17): 37–40

9

The development of a standardised approach to wound care in ICU

Janet L Hadcock

Reflection and evaluation of wound care administered within the intensive care unit where the author is based suggested that an inadequate level of care was being provided. No structured approach existed; documentation was poor, with practitioners struggling to make decisions on appropriate care. A research study supported these reflections, and implied that wound care was delivered on an ad hoc basis. Results indicated that this was due to the limited knowledge base of practitioners in relation to the wound healing process, and wound management. Few staff had ever received any training on this topic and most knowledge was acquired through trial and error. No evidence-based approach to wound care was in place: thus, care was random and outdated. The results from the research study stimulated the development of a comprehensive evidence-based reference guide on the topic of wound care, which was designed for use in the clinical setting, and has allowed the development of a structured approach to wound care.

The critical care nurse is primarily involved in caring for the critically ill patient, and wound care is often a long way down the list of priorities within intensive care. Initially this is understandable for resuscitation of the critically ill, but if holistic nursing care is to be provided wound management is important and must be addressed (Malone, 1992).

Over the past decade, the management of patients with wounds has received much attention. Until the early 1980s there was little understanding of wound management, and for many nurses the area was enshrouded in ritualistic mystique that included the use of forceps, masks, gowns and strict aseptic technique (Bale, 1993). Today, the bewildering array of wound care products on the market can serve to confuse rather than inform nurses working in the clinical area and can lead to inconsistent approaches to wound care (Turner, 1991).

The location for this small study was a nine-bedded general adult intensive care unit (ICU) within an acute teaching hospital. There was no standardised approach to wound management, and nurses based the wound care provided on clinical experience, gut instinct, and tradition, rather than sound clinically supported/appropriate evidence. Therefore, wound care was not measurable, sometimes erratic, and often not research based. Reflection on practice highlighted how a dressing was often applied by one nurse, only to be removed by the following nurse, as he/she believed that a different course of treatment was best. The patient was not receiving a quality service, and improvements needed to be made (Department of Health [DoH], 1993). The development of a standardised approach to wound care was a step towards providing an optimum level of evidence-based practice, against which actual performance could be compared (DoH, 1998).

Literature review

Because of various factors it is thought that approximately 40% of critically ill intensive care patients develop pressure sores (Bergstrom *et al*, 1987), which need to be assessed and documented regularly to facilitate appropriate management. Wound assessment charts are a means of outlining the severity of breaks in skin continuity, and can monitor the healing process. If such tools are not used documentation of wound management remains poor, which can slow healing, despite the legal and professional implications for nurses (Sterling, 1996).

In this ICU a wound assessment chart was available but infrequently used, perhaps because of an inadequate knowledge base hindering assessment (Hon and Jones, 1996). Tapp (1990) suggests that many nurses prioritise hands-on care over documentation, but if documentation about the wound remains poor, continuity of care and rationale are lost which might lead to the fragmented application of different dressing products and slow wound healing (Carroll and Johnson, 1991).

Other studies have indicated that nurses provide poor wound management due to inadequate knowledge. Koh (1993) carried out a small survey to investigate whether nurses kept up-to-date with current knowledge, practice, theory and research about wound healing. This was undertaken on two medical and two surgical wards in a London teaching hospital. Results demonstrated that all respondents had some knowledge about certain aspects of wound healing; however, much knowledge appeared superficial and incomplete.

The assumption that experience enhances knowledge was found to be inaccurate and, in fact, the reverse was true. The reasons for this were unclear and it has been suggested that it may be due to a theory/practice gap (O'Connor, 1993), or a lack of sound knowledge on this topic (Guilding, 1993). These authors believe that more education, linked to a strong evidence base, is necessary to transform wound management from the current 'hit and miss' process.

Nurses today are increasingly concerned with ethical, political and economic questions that directly affect patient care. Nursing is essentially a practical discipline (Hawkett, 1990), but practice without a theoretical basis becomes ritualised performance (Kershaw, 1986). Nursing journals contain an abundance of information on the concept and practice of wound healing, yet some nurses continue with outdated practices. With the advent of specialist tissue viability nurses (Russell, 2000) who have specialised knowledge that can be disseminated to their peers, nurses have established their own distinct body of knowledge pertaining to this topic.

Nurses' autonomy also seems to play a part in wound management. A study by Flanagan (1992b) of twenty-four qualified nurses found that relationships with medical staff could influence dressing selection. She found that nurses from medical areas were more likely to be responsible for the selection of wound dressings than colleagues within surgical environments. She also noted that nurses in intensive care were found to be more autonomous, and conflicts between medical staff were less likely. The explanation for this view suggested that some medical staff viewed ICU nurses as specialists in all areas of nursing, including wound care, pain management and bereavement care, because they work in an intensive care environment and provide care on a 1:1 ratio.

This was only a small-scale survey and experience levels were not mentioned, but perhaps the ICU nurses involved had more managerial experience — hence more autonomy. Malone (1992) disagrees with Flanagan (1992b) about wound care and ICU nurses, as she believes that they have much to learn about this topic. McSharry (1995) suggested that nurses are professionals in their own field and they wish to be guided by specialists to improve the care they provide.

It seems to be generally accepted in the available literature that to make an appropriate choice of dressing, it is necessary to have an understanding of the healing process, and how that process may be supported and enhanced (Koh, 1993). The literature appears to suggest that nurses need to be updated not only on available dressings and their uses, but also on the healing and assessment process (Flanagan, 1992b). Most of the research on this topic has been done on a small scale, making it difficult to generalise. Further study is required to investigate the gaps in skills and allow education programmes to be developed which will make the decisions on dressing selection more logical and scientific.

Method

The research undertaken aimed to establish the criteria which influence nurses when selecting dressings for superficial pressure sores. A descriptive survey design was used to collect qualitative data (Polit and Hungler, 1993) through a confidential questionnaire that asked two closed questions and eight open-ended questions (Oppenhiem, 1992). Stratified random sampling (Cormack, 1996) was used to gain a sample of twenty nurses at grades D to G, from the total population of forty-three nurses within this ICU. Sixty-five per cent (n=13) of the questionnaires were completed and returned.

The completed questionnaires were transcribed to ensure handwriting was not recognised, which also made them easier to read. Reading and rereading allowed the researcher to become immersed in the data. Different colour pens were used to highlight initial themes, which (with short notes) are referred to as 'open-coding' (Berg, 1989). Unrelated data were eliminated (Field and Morse, 1985) allowing the information to be collapsed into similar but broader categories. Efforts were made to maintain the richness of the original data by not compressing the results too much and using original questionnaires for clarity (Polit and Hungler, 1993).

Once initial coding had been undertaken, an independent practitioner was invited to organise replies, without having access to the categories generated by the researcher. The final lists were discussed and minor adjustments made to the final coding, thus increasing internal validity. Transcripts were then reread along with final categories, to ensure that they covered all aspects of the content.

It is acknowledged that the small size of the sample does not allow the results to be generalised, but this was unavoidable as the study was undertaken in the researcher's own time in an effort to investigate local practices. This should not detract from the importance of the findings, which show that ICU nurses' knowledge of wound management has still not improved even though previous studies showed similar results (Flanagan, 1992b; Koh, 1993).

Results

The results indicated that only five respondents had received any formal education on wound care as student nurses, which was based on the concept of aseptic technique. A further five had received formal education on this topic once qualified, but the basis of this training was product presentation by company representatives and not wound management. These results are supported by published work that found a lack of sound in-depth knowledge on this topic, which may be the root cause why current wound management is based on trial and error or tradition (Koh, 1993; O'Connor, 1993).

The educational framework for wound management appeared to be inept or absent for all grades of staff, as any education had revolved around aseptic technique and individual dressing products, rather than the concept of wound management as a whole. The overwhelming view from nurses participating in this study suggested that they did not know enough about the topic.

The knowledge base of both current D-grade staff nurses and experienced G-grade sisters (some with over ten years clinical practice) was poor. This suggested that education on this topic had not improved or progressed over the last ten years in this clinical area, and perhaps explains why experience of this topic remains superficial and incomplete (Koh, 1993). The knowledge base of staff appeared to be similar throughout the grades, thus implying that experience did not improve knowledge or practice within this one area.

While all nurses defined a necrotic sore correctly, and 84.5% (n=11) defined a superficial pressure sore correctly, definitions of granulating and epithelialising wounds were poor/inaccurate. All stated that they found wound assessment difficult in practice, yet if appropriate wound care is to be provided, accurate wound assessment is fundamental (Flanagan, 1997).

The respondents listed various factors that influenced their choice of dressing product (*Table 9.1*). The dressings in stock played a large part in the decision-making process of these nurses, which may not have been the most appropriate method of dressing selection. The results suggested that once accurate assessment had taken place, a methodical approach was required to assist the decision-making process on dressing selection. This needed to simplify the difficult choice of which dressing to choose, while informing the practitioner on its structure and correct usage.

Table 9.1: Factors which influence dressing selection	
Factors	**No. of respondents**
Resources available/dressings in stock	6
Patient comfort/position of sore	6
Frequency of dressing change/time needed to change it	5
Knowledge/previous experience	4
Influence from others, colleagues, medical staff, hospital policies	3
Effect of dressing on surrounding healthy skin	2
Stability of patient for turning/moving	2
Cost of dressings	2
Don't know	1

Seven of the respondents did not feel that the wound care they provided was evidence-based, but described it as personal preference, which ultimately means ritualistic care (Flanagan, 1992a). Most felt it was the responsibility of 'others' to keep themselves abreast of new research, but they could not identify who these 'others' were or who updated them (Turner, 1991). The lack of evidence-based care was highlighted when the respondents reviewed the standard of wound care currently being provided: four replies indicated a good standard of practice while seven disagreed. The respondents felt that conflicting opinions and lack of standardisation made the current level of wound care poor, and offered poor continuity of patient care.

Practice development

The results indicated that nurses were not assessing wounds as well as they should have been, therefore highlighting a need for further training to develop knowledge and skills. It is important to consider the condition of the patient as well as the wound if holistic care is to be provided. Nurses need to be aware that critically ill patients' wounds do not always heal at a normal rate; this is usually because of their physiological condition and is not always the result of poor wound management (Collins, 1996). It was apparent that to improve the wound care provided in this area, nurses needed to develop their knowledge base, standardise the care provided, and strive towards the goal of improving the general condition of critically ill patients.

Education programme

A comprehensive reference guide was developed to respond to the needs of intensive care nurses. This covered a multitude of topics which aimed to develop the knowledge base of practitioners, so they could make informed evidence-based decisions about wound management. This was named the 'Wound care reference guide', and contained information on the topics listed in *Table 9.2*.

To introduce this guide, and ensure it was useful and relevant to nurses, there needed to be a multi-method approach. A combination of formal and informal teaching sessions, along with practical demonstrations, supported and explained the information presented within the guide. As approximately forty nurses work within this ICU, the education process took several months, but this was necessary to change the current culture of wound management within this area. Once they had understood the concept of wound healing and the assessment strategy, the nurses began to use this package in practice.

Table 9.2: Information in the 'Wound care reference guide'
The structure and function of skin
Phases of wound healing
Local factors affecting wound healing
External factors affecting wound healing
How to conduct accurate wound assessment
Documentation of wounds
Goals of wound healing
Review of products currently available within intensive care, including product structure, function, tips on usage, along with manufacturers' information
Glossary
References

Utilised in the practice setting, the guidelines facilitate a systematic assessment and documentation of the wound. They contain wound photographs demonstrating the physical differences in tissue found on the wound floor, eg. necrotic, sloughy, granulating. This assists the assessment process, and enables practitioners to determine the amount and kind of tissue on the wound floor and to complete the wound assessment chart correctly (*Figure 9.1*). The assessment strategy also collects information on:

- size of wound
- amount and type of exudate
- odour
- condition of wound margins
- any signs of infection.

The guide will teach the user about the goals of wound healing, wound management products, as well as guidance on how to use them correctly and efficiently. By clearly directing and guiding the nurse through the decision-making process, the reference guide empowers a higher standard of patient care by providing evidence to support the decision-making process.

Patient's name _____	Date _____	Date _____	Date_____
_____	Type of wound _____	Type of wound _____	Type of wound_____
Hospital no _____	_____	_____	_____
Unit no _____	Location _____	Location _____	Location_____
_____	_____	_____	_____
Wound dimensions	Max width _____mm	Max width _____ mm	Max width _____ mm
	Max length _____mm	Max length _____ mm	Max length _____mm
	Max depth _____mm	Max depth _____ mm	Max depth _____ mm
Sketch wound shape			
Grade of wound	Stage _____	Stage _____	Stage _____
Per cent of tissue on the wound floor	Healthy granulation ____%	Healthy granulation ____ %	Healthy granulation____ %
	Slough _____%	Slough_____ %	Slough _____%
	Necrotic _____%	Necrotic_____%	Necrotic_____%
Exudate/discharge	Colour _____	Colour _____	Colour _____
	Consistency _____	Consistency _____	Consistency _____
	Amount _____	Amount _____	Amount _____
Odour	None/some/offensive _____	None/some/offensive _____	None/some/offensive _____
Wound edges	Colour _____	Colour _____	Colour _____
	Oedema present yes/no ___	Oedema present yes/no ___	Oedema present yes/no ___
Surrounding skin condition	Blanching erythema _____	Blanching erythema _____	Blanching erythema _____
	Non-blanching erythema ___	Non-blanching erythema ___	Non-blanching erythema___
	Wet or dry _____	Wet or dry _____	Wet or dry _____
	Oedema present yes/no ____	Oedema present yes/no ____	Oedema present yes/no ____
Infection	Suspected yes/no _____	Suspected yes/no _____	Suspected yes/no _____
	Wound swab	Wound swab	Wound swab
	sent _____	sent _____	sent_____
	Organism isolated	Organism isolated	Organism isolated
	_____	_____	_____
Dressing schedule:			
Proposed review date:	_____	_____	_____
Wound assessed by:			

Figure 9.1: Wound assessment chart

How this works in practice

A detailed description of the wound is formulated, which is imperative to achieve appropriate dressing selection (Flanagan, 1997). *Figure 9.2* demonstrates how the reference guide works in practice. It was planned to incorporate a wound dressing formulary into the 'Wound care reference guide', but during its development the trust launched its own formulary and dressing guidelines. No education process accompanied their distribution and they were not widely disseminated; therefore, practitioners within this area did not use this tool.

This may have been due to the lack of knowledge in relation to wound care, as the formulary did not address the knowledge base deficits believed to be present on the concept of wound management as a whole. The lack of information about this tool may have caused practitioners to view it as yet another poster by a wound care company promoting its products within the clinical setting. Therefore, the dressing guidelines contained in the formulary were incorporated into the reference guide, allowing the trust's wound care formulary to be used appropriately.

When the extent of wound damage had been been assessed, it was recorded using the assessment chart developed within ICU. The type of tissue on the wound bed, along with the amount of exudate allows an appropriate decision to be made on the right type of dressing product. The formulary is consulted and provides the name of a suitable generic type of dressing for the particular type of wound. A key at the bottom converts these generic terms into individual product brands, available within this area.

The reference guide provides independent information on these dressing products, their structure and function along with tips on use. This information makes it easy to use the right dressing on the right wound, at the right time and in the right way. Manufacturers' information and evidence for practice is also provided, along with an example of the product, allowing the nurse to become knowledgeable about the product selected before use. The 'Wound care reference guide' is kept at a central location within the ICU and is frequently used at the patient's bedside facilitating more accurate wound assessment.

Step 1	The wound is assessed, utilising knowledge about the healing process and assessment, from the 'Wound care reference guide', eg. infected, heavily exuding wound

Wound care formulary consulted. Look along infected wound line until box labelled 'high level of exudate' is reached. This will demonstrate recommended primary and secondary dressings, and one each will be selected, eg. Primary: activated charcoal cloth with silver, hydro-fibre or alginate; Secondary: absorbent pads, hydropolymer, foam	**Step 2**

Step 3	Dressing key at bottom of wound care formulary consulted to determine product names, eg. Primary: Actisorb, Aquacel, Kaltostat; Secondary: postoperative pad, Tielle, Lyofoam

A review of these products can be found at the back of the 'Wound care reference guide', with recommendation on their use. It is recommended that this be used to ensure products are used correctly, thus providing quality, cost-effective care	**Step 4**

Figure 9.2: The 'Wound care reference guide' in use

Conclusion

The package has been in place for ten months, and reflection on practice indicates that nurses within this area are using the reference guide regularly at the patient's bedside. It is suggested that this structured approach is improving practice within this area allowing informed, evidence-based quality care to be provided. Because of the nature of wounds and patients cared for, a degree of flexibility is still required to address individual needs in special circumstances.

The impact that this comprehensive reference guide has had on the level of wound care within the ICU environment needs to be measured, and then reported and disseminated. It is planned to repeat the research which stimulated the creation of the reference guide in twelve months. It is anticipated that nurses will now have a better understanding of the concept of wound care, and a greater insight into and access to the necessary support/resources available.

Although this reference guide was designed for use within one ICU, it has been acknowledged that its principles could be utilised in other areas. Various directorates within the trust are awaiting evaluation, and are interested in using this pack in the future. The reference guide is now utilised within the tissue viability core competency which is part of the Greater Manchester Multi-Professional Critical Care Programme. This is a collaborative venture including thirteen acute Trusts, and the private sector.

Key points

❖ The research suggested that there is an inadequate knowledge base on the concept of wound management within the intensive care environment.

❖ The results stimulated the development of a standardised evidence-based approach to wound management.

❖ Quality wound care can only be provided if the staff involved have a comprehensive knowledge base on the whole concept of wound management.

Reference

Bale S (1993) Wound assessment. *Surg Nurse* **6**(1): 11–14

Berg BL (1989) *Qualitative Research Methods for the Social Sciences*. Allyn and Bacon, New York

Bergstrom N, Demuth PJ, Braden BJ (1987) A clinical trial of the Braden Scale for predicting pressure sore risk. *Nurse Clinician* **22**: 417–28

Carroll R, Johnson L (1991) Using a wound assessment chart. *Nurs Standard* **5**(25): 8–9

Collins CM (1996) Nutrition and wound healing. *Care Critically Ill* **12**(3): 87–90

Cormack DFS (1996) *The Research Process in Nursing*. 3rd edn. Blackwell Scientific, Oxford

Department of Health (1993) *Pressure Sores — A Key Quality Indicator*. HMSO, London

Department of Health (1998) *Our Healthier Nation: A Contract for Health*. HMSO, London

Field PA, Morse JM (1985) *Nursing Research: The Application of Qualitative Approaches*. Croom Helm, London

Flanagan M (1992a) Variables influencing nurses' selection of wound dressings. *J Wound Care* **1**(1): 33–43

Flanagan M (1992b) Outside influences. *Nurs Times* **88**(36): 72–8

Flanagan M (1997) A practical framework for wound assessment 2: methods. *Br J Nurs* **6**(1): 6–11

Guilding L (1993) Dimensions of nursing knowledge in wound care. *Br J Nurs* **2**(14): 712–16

Hawkett S (1990) A gap which must be bridged: nurses' attitudes to theory and practice. *Prof Nurse* **6**(3): 166–72

Hon J, Jones C (1996) The documentation of wounds in an acute hospital setting. *Br J Nurs* **5**(17): 1040–5

Kershaw B (1986) *Models for Nursing*. John Wiley, Chichester

Koh S (1993) Dressing practices. *Nurs Times* **89**(42): 82–6

McSharry M (1995) The evolving role of the clinical nurse specialist. *Br J Nurs* **4**(11): 641–6

Malone C (1992) Intensive pressures. *Nurs Times* **88**(36): 57–62

O'Connor H (1993) Bridging the gap. *Nurs Times* **89**(32): 63–6

Oppenheim AN (1992) *Questionnaire Design, Interviewing and Attitude Measurement*. Pinter Publishers, London

Polit DF, Hungler BP (1993) *Essentials of Nursing Research: Methods, Appraisal and Utilization*. 3rd edn. JB Lippincott Co, Philadelphia

Russell L (2000) Understanding physiology of wound healing and how dressings help. *Br J Nurs* **9**(1): 10–21

Sterling C (1996) Methods of wound assessment documentation: a study. *Nurs Standard* **11**(10): 38–41

Tapp RA (1990) Inhibitors and facilitators to documentation of nursing practice. *Western J Nurs Res* **12**(2): 229–40

Turner TD (1982) Which dressing and why. *Nurs Times* **78**(29): 41–4

Turner V (1991) Standardization of wound care. *Nurs Standard* **5**(19): 25–8

Section IV:
Practice

10

The importance of wound documentation and classification

Linda Russell

Good wound documentation has become increasingly important over the last ten years. Wound assessment provides a baseline situation against which a patient's plan of care can be evaluated. A number of documents have been implemented including the *Code of Professional Conduct for Nurses, Midwives and Health Visitors* (UKCC, 1992), the *Post-registration Education Project* (UKCC, 1997), *Standards of Records and Record Keeping* (UKCC, 1998), and *Keeping the Record Straight* (NHS Executive [NHS E], 1993). These documents require nurses to maintain their professional knowledge and competence, and to recognise any deficiency in their knowledge. Having recognised any deficiency they should read the relevant literature and/or attend a study day on wound care. Nursing records are the first source of evidence investigated when a complaint is made. Wound assessment is very complex and a standardised approach to evaluation needs to be adopted. Such evaluation should encompass colour classification, wound measurement, and classification of tissue type present in the wound. There are numerous methods of measuring wounds; these range from the simple, such as manual estimation by means of a ruler or wound tracing, to the more technical procedures, eg. computer, image analysis, and colour imaging using hue saturation and intensity. Photography, in conjunction with nursing notes, provides a very good form of wound documentation and can provide clear evidence if required for legal cases.

The management of wounds became a nursing responsibility in the 1930s when experienced ward sisters were trained to change dressings. Gradually, this role grew and became a nursing responsibility (Dealey, 1994). Over the last ten years the emphasis on good wound documentation has increased due to an increase in the number of wound care products available and the increased likelihood of litigation cases.

Accurate, holistic, wound assessment needs to be made by the practitioner which requires many skills. Dealey (1994) states that the ability to make an accurate assessment of the patient's wound is considered to be an important nursing skill. Holistic wound assessment provides a baseline case upon which to focus the plan of care, set relevant goals, and apply relevant wound care products to promote healing (Briggs and Banks, 1995; Williams, 1997).

Inferior wound assessment can result in inappropriate wound management and consequently lead to increased costs in nursing time, use of products, and patient suffering (Williams, 1997). In the past, nurses have not employed evidence-based nursing practice but employed anecdotal evidence. However, in recent years this has started to change and nurses now challenge old ritualistic care.

Nurses are required to document the progress of wounds and an assessment form is a useful method of documentation (Morison, 1992; Dealey, 1994). Morison (1992) states that accurate observation of wounds can be made easy by the use of a chart that highlights the factors needing consideration when wounds are being assessed. These also serve as an aid in teaching student nurses.

Accurate documentation of wound characteristics enables comparison of the wound assessment by the nurse involved in patient care (Benbow, 1995). Correct wound assessment is dependent on an understanding of the physiology of wound healing, the factors that delay the process, and the optimal conditions required at the wound surface to maximise healing (Flanagan, 1996; Kerstein, 1997). A holistic approach to wound management needs to be employed in order to monitor the rate of healing and the effectiveness of planned care at promoting healing. Wound assessment is problematic as it is very subjective and only as good as the practitioner undertaking the assessment. Therefore, if the practitioner's knowledge is deficient in the stages of wound healing, they may be unable to correctly identify the wound status (Flanagan, 1996) and the consequence may be an inappropriate dressing selection.

The UKCC's (1992) *Code of Professional Conduct* and *Post-registration Education Project* (UKCC, 1997) pronounce that the nurse must 'take every opportunity to develop and maintain his or her professional knowledge and competence'. Nurses have a duty to attend study days and read relevant literature where they consider their own knowledge is deficient. However, nurses may have to undertake study in their own time and often have to finance courses themselves.

Morison (1992) and Bennett and Moody (1995) state the importance of maintaining clear, concise, nursing records. Failure to do so can be seen as a negligent act and a breach of nurses' duty of care. An agreed, nationally applied system of wound assessment forms would provide a useful framework and assist in documentation. Since no pressure sore grading system has been nationally agreed this may be some time in coming.

Only one small study on the documenting of wound management has been undertaken (Briggs and Banks, 1995). This involved 120 patients with 152 wounds being treated at a teaching hospital in Leeds. All wounds, which included pressure sores, leg ulcers and infected wounds, required healing by secondary intention, and were graded on the Association of Enterostomal Therapists' (1987) grading system. If a patient had pressure sore damage of 2–4, then the nursing care plan was reviewed for evidence related to the treatment of the pressure sore. The first review revealed that in nursing records only 56.2% of patients had a specific care plan outlining treatment for pressure damage. In 27.4% of cases the care plan made no mention of pressure damage, or no plan of care for pressure damage had been devised, and there was no evidence of pressure sore treatment in 16.4% of cases.

Consequently, a working group was set up to develop new wound care guidelines and a documentation form was designed based on Morison (1992) and Dealey (1994). An audit was repeated with a sample of 136 patients with 152 wounds. Great improvement had occurred and 99% of patients had a designated care plan. The assessment appeared to be more thorough when the new wound assessment form was used, as it made information available at a glance. However, the follow-up audit on the new documentation demonstrated that the first assessment was completed very fully, but reassessments were completed very poorly with regard to dressing changes and renewals.

This study clearly demonstrated that nurses completed the wound assessment form but did not understand the importance of reassessment and accurate record keeping as advocated by the UKCC's (1998) *Guidelines for Records and Record Keeping* and the NHS Executive's (NHS E's) *Keeping the Record Straight* (1993). Nursing records are the first source of evidence investigated when a complaint is made. Nurses need to keep this in mind when documenting. Hammersley and Atkinson (1991) state that nursing records produce a documentary description of the patient's stay in hospital and the nursing record is considered to be a concrete display of professional competence.

The indices for wound assessment and classification encompass many characteristics, eg. wound classification, wound size, wound edges, under-mining, type of tissue present in the wound, exudate, and condition of surrounding tissue (Hampton, 1997).

The healing process is a complex mechanism and conceivably this is why no standardised approach has ever been adopted. Flanagan (1997) suggests that if a standardised approach could be adopted it would allow competent understanding for all practitioners, easy comparisons for wound evaluation, accurate documentation, and ultimately provide the patient with cost-effective wound care and reduce suffering resulting from the wound. In America, the National Pressure Ulcer Advisory Panel (1989) and the Agency for Health published guidelines for prevention and treatment of pressure sores. The Wound Healing Society published guidelines for assessment of wounds and evaluation of healing (Lazarus and Cooper, 1994). Gentzkow (1995) commented that the guidelines were deficient in clarity on how to assess wound healing during clinical investigations.

Wound classification

Several methods of classifying wounds exist (Cuzzell, 1988; Healey, 1995; Xakellis and Frantz, 1997). The literature reviewed has not revealed the existence of an international, or even a national, wound classification system. The classification of a wound depends on the practitioner's knowledge of skin physiology (Flanagan, 1997). Direct observation is the most widespread method of assessing and classifying wounds. The colour and characteristics of the wound surface are indicative of certain types of wound (Cuzzell, 1988). Buntinx and

Beckers (1996) argue that this approach is oversimplified; however, in reality it is easy and quick to use and has no cost implications.

Some practitioners, such as Torrance (1983) and Shea (1975), advocate the use of a stage system to define wounds. However, Xakellis and Frantz (1997) state that the staging system initially works well for ulcer assessment, but is inappropriate for long-term assessment of healing. 'Pressure ulcers do not heal in reverse stages' (Maklebust, 1995). For example, a stage 4 ulcer does not also progress to stage 3 and subsequently through stages 2 to 1. Pressure sores heal through a process of granulation, wound contraction, epithelialisation and scar formation (Xakellis and Frantz, 1997).

Xakellis and Frantz (1997) reviewed three strategies developed by clinical experts: the Agency for Health Care Policy (Bergstrom and Bennett, 1994), the Research Wound Healing Society (Lazarus and Cooper, 1994) and the Pressure Sore Status Tool (Bates-Jenson *et al*, 1992). The three groups recommended certain measures (*Table 10.1*) which were taken from the empirical evidence supporting effectiveness. These measures represent expert opinion regarding the clinical monitoring of the important changes that occur during ulcer healing. Unfortunately, the eleven points may not fulfil all practitioners' needs. Furthermore, not all the measures will necessarily be required to assess an ulcer.

Table 10.1: Clinical measures recommended for monitoring ulcer healing	
Wound factors	Size/area
	Stage/depth
	Location
	Shape
	Exudate
	Necrotic tissue
	Granulation
	Epithelialisation
	Sinus
	Skin edges/undermining
	Erythema/skin colour
	Induration
Surrounding skin factors	Erythema/skin colour
	Induration

Adapted from Xakellis and Frantz, 1997

The wound classification procedure commonly employed in England is that of the pink, red, yellow, green and black system, initially launched in the mid-1970s by a company called Lederle. Lederle recommended that Varidase was indicated for use on necrotic wounds and used a colour system for identifying wounds in its promotional literature. This system was then adopted by the Wound Care Society in 1988 (Flanagan, 1992) and is still the most common method used in practice and for teaching purposes (*Table 10.2*). Flanagan (1997) suggests using a classification model based on the clinical appearance of the wound and the requirements for the promotion of wound healing. Research is required to discover how nurses actually classify wounds in clinical practice.

Table 10.2: Wound classification
Pink
This is healthy tissue in the final stages of healing. Pinky white epithelial tissue migrates from the wound edges and the tissue will contain remnants of hair follicle in the dermis (Flanagan, 1997; Hampton, 1997).
Red
This tissue is deep red or pink and has raised uneven red granules giving the tissue a 'beefy appearance'. Fine capillary loops have been laid down and consequently this tissue can bleed easily. Hohn and Pounce (1977) state that unnecessary cleansing of granulating wounds can cause more harm and it is more beneficial to maintain the optimum environment for healing.
Green
Collier (1994) states that green exudate does not always indicate clinical infection as bacteria can colonise in wounds without harming the host. However, green exudate may demonstrate that *Pseudomonas* spp. are present in the wound bed. Pathogenic organisms can delay wound healing and the wound may demonstrate signs of clinical infection such as inflammation. Exudates from clinically infected wounds range from yellow, green, dark red/brown or grey (Hampton, 1997). Where an infection is suspected, a swab should be taken to identify the organism causing the infection.
Yellow
This tissue comprises the remnants of dead cells from the wound surface. The debris contains large amounts of dead leucocytes, bacteria, and fibrous tissue, and these give the tissue a yellow creamy appearance. Flanagan (1977) states that slough is a natural part of healing, but does necessitate rehydration with a hydrogel. The presence of slough should not be taken as an indicator that the wound is not healthy, but that the wound is removing dead tissue to make way for healthy tissue.
Black
This tissue comprises hard black/brown leathery eschar. Xakellis and Chrischilles (1992) demonstrated that necrotic tissue at baseline was associated with slower healing times. This tissue has to be debrided before any wound healing can take place. The quickest method of debridement is surgical, but usually requires an anaesthetic. Conservative measures are rehydration of the tissue by scoring the tissue with a blade and allowing the hydrogel to hydrate the leathery tissue. Another method, which has gained in popularity, is biological larvae therapy (maggots) (Hampton, 1997).

Wound assessment and measurements

Regardless of which wound assessment model is employed, the case history should be carefully studied to determine how long the wound has been present, its location, the state of the surrounding skin, and whether any undermining and tracking is present. Other factors, extrinsic and intrinsic, have to be examined, as these will also delay wound healing (Hampton, 1997). The final picture is gained when size, colour and measurement of the wound have been obtained; only then can a plan of care be made.

When assessing a wound, measurements must always be taken the same way (length and width in centimetres) with a tape measure. To increase reliability of results always measure the largest and widest aspects of the wound or measure from head-to-toe and side-to-side of the wound (Cooper, 1992). For the practitioner to decide if effective wound care is being applied, measurements need to be taken to evaluate the wound's progress. Van Rijswijk and Polansky's (1994) study demonstrated that:

There appears to be sufficient evidence to suggest that weeks of ineffective treatment modalities can be avoided if appropriate clinical assessments are performed at least once a week.

The patient needs to be examined on the same side and in the same position at each assessment to enable precise documentation (Melhuish and Plassmann, 1994; Bates-Jensen, 1995; Plassmann, 1995).

A wound area is normally measured two-dimensionally by multiplying length and width of the wound; however, it may be measured in a more complex and accurate way. Methods of measuring a wound vary from very sophisticated methods, such as photography, planimetry, or computer imaging, to less sophisticated methods such as tracing on acetate. Volume, which is three-dimensional, is estimated by the length, width and depth measurement or may be measured by casts or sterophotography, magnetic resonance imaging, or ultrasound. These methods tend to be employed for research projects to detect detailed changes in the wound but this procedure is both complex and costly.

Wound tracing

The most popular and cheapest method of assessment is by tracing on to transparent sheets marked with a grid which is then transferred to graph paper, or placing the traced acetate directly in the patient's notes (Plassmann, 1995). Transparencies tend to be more accessible on wards and this may be the reason why it is the method preferred by nurses. Additionally, it is the least time consuming of the methods mentioned above. This method, as it is dependent upon the observer being able to define the wound edges, is very subjective and depends on clinical judgement (Ramirez *et al*, 1969; Majeske, 1992; Flanagan, 1997). Despite this, it is the most commonly taught method in the classroom, and it is far better to have some documentation rather than none. Measurements of wounds should be encouraged as it is an integral part of the assessment tool and must be recorded, as it is important for medicolegal reasons (Moody, 1993).

Wound tracing does have its limitations in that wounds are three-dimensional and tracing gives no information regarding the depth of the wound. If this information is recorded separately the tracing will provide an overall evaluation of how the wound is progressing (Flanagan, 1997). Anthony (1987) suggests that wound tracing is less reliable with regard to interobserver error. It was demonstrated that the tracing method was unreliable when the longest and shortest measurements were repeated by different interobservers. The best way to overcome this problem is to have the identical observer enabling the same method to be employed. However, Anthony (1987) demonstrated that different observers obtain different readings of computer measurements of pressure sores. This was attributed to a number of reasons such as the criteria used to decide where the edge of the wound was, and different tracing techniques.

Various methods of evaluating wound tracing have been undertaken such as tracing the wound and then counting the number of grid squares covering the wound (Gowland Hopkins and Jamieson, 1983), tracing the wound areas on to acetate sheet and then cutting the shape out and weighing it (Crisculob and Oldfield, 1988). Sterophotogrammetry is used to measure rates of healing (Bulstrode and Goode, 1986) and involves the use of two cameras simultaneously. These two photographs are then analysed using a stero-comparator which produces a three-dimensional picture by combining the photographs (Anthony, 1987). All of these methods are very time-consuming but have proved to be accurate.

Kundin (1985) designed a gauge which measures length and width of a wound in one single measurement. In 1989, he produced the empirical formula, shown below, that assumes a wound is irregular in shape and that only 75% of the wound's squared area can be calculated using the gauge method:

Area of the wound = length x breadth x 0.75

Thomas and Wysocki (1990) demonstrated a correlation between the gauge, acetate tracing, and photograph systems of measuring wounds. The Kundin ruler was found to underestimate the wound area by several orders of magnitude (Plassmann, 1995). The gauge systems set the standard for the measurements of wounds, despite the fact that they are the least reliable method and give a high standard deviation, making the system unacceptable for research trials.

Computers and wound measurements

Over the last ten years the use of computers has increased considerably, particularly in wound measurement. A tracing of the wound can be transferred to a computer and the image analysed automatically (Brohannan and Pfaller, 1983; Anthony, 1987; Majeske, 1992; Ahroni *et al*, 1993). Palmer *et al* (1989) used a camera linked to a computer to measure wound area. However, it was discovered that a camera angle of 200 to the perpendicular resulted in a reduction of the measured area by approximately 10%. Thus, care must be taken to standardise photography technique.

Computer analysis is a simple and reliable way to measure wounds accurately and reproducibly. It has proved far more reliable than manual measure-ments, which have been shown to have as much as 25% variation on repeat estimations between observers; computer measurements have been shown to be associated with a less than 0.2% deviation on remeasurement (Mekkes and Westerhof, 1992). Current data suggest that measuring the ulcer's dimensions, exudate, and predominant tissue will provide the most valid indicators for monitoring the change in pressure ulcers over time. One of the major problems with trying to measure a wound is the natural curvature of the body; this is due to the fact that all the tools used for measurement are designed to measure wounds as a flat object; consequently, they will be inaccurate (Plassmann, 1995).

Using five volunteers, three of whom were male and two of whom were female, four of whom were right-handed and one of whom was left-handed, Taylor (1997) studied various shapes, ie. circles, rectangles, and polygons, traced by a computer program — 'mouseyes'. A mouse was used to trace image outline, which was then stored on to the personal computer. The program was designed to digitise the perimeter of an image and then calculate the surface area within it, and also to calculate the linear distances between features within an image.

The results demonstrated that this system's accuracy was associated with a 1.3% error (which was less than Taylor's [1995] studies, which had a 2% error). This work highlighted problems with shapes of less than $1cm^2$. Taylor suggests that magnification would solve this problem. Several measurements had to be taken but this was not always practical with the patients enlisted for research. Angular shapes posed particular problems, as their straight sides needed to be aligned with the vertical and horizontal axes. Further work is required to improve the system so that it is more accurate and reproducible.

Melhuish and Plassmann (1994) investigated fourteen patients, seven with pilonidal sinus excision and seven with abdominal wound cavities after surgical procedures. Wounds were evaluated at weekly intervals using structured light measurements for the area, volume and depth. The wound edges were highlighted with a mouse, and the computer calculated the number of pixels in the area being studied. Results demonstrated a correlation between volume and circumference using the Gilman (1990) formula to standardise the measurements. One criticism cited by Melhuish and Plassman (1994) is the problem of measuring the area and volume with any degree of exactness due to the location of the wound. As a result of the correlation between wound circumference, wound area, and wound volume, it is possible to monitor a wound's progress by measuring the circumference.

Hue saturation and intensity

Hue saturation and intensity (HSI) analysis perceives colour using a similar mechanism to the human eye. Colour is specified using measurements of three primary colours, just as the eye does using nervous impulses from colour-specific rods and cones. Hue measures the wavelength of the main colour. Saturation is the amount of white light included within the colour, and intensity is a measure of brightness. The HSI components are independent, so any change in brightness or contrast of the original image results in a change of a single HSI component. Thus, any changes between/within wounds can be seen easily and quantified.

No studies exist on using HSI for measurement and classification of pressure sores. Boardman and Melhuish (1994) studied ten patients with pilonidal excision and abdominal wound and groin abscesses. Eight patients healed normally and two had wound infections which were confirmed with positive cultures. Various infected wounds were studied, including abdominal wounds, groin abscesses, and pilonidal excisions. Healing was measured using image analysis which demonstrated that HSI analysis provides an improved means of identifying wound areas. The authors demonstrated that subtle changes in the continuous percentage hue colour traces can indicate problems with the wound.

A recent study on a burns patient using colour imaging discovered a high correlation between wound severity and HSI at five to seven days. It was concluded that this method could be used for tracking wound severity in a clinical setting (Hansen *et al*, 1997).

Wound depth

The depth of a wound can by measured in a number of ways, eg. using sophisticated sterophotography, ultrasonic scanning and probing the wound with a swab, and examination with gloved finger (Krasner, 1992; Plassmann, 1995; Flanagan, 1997). Techniques employed in research are unsuitable for the clinical setting and everyday use (Franz and Johnson, 1992; Gentzkow, 1995). Dimensions of a deep wound should be measured using a cotton tipped applicator to enable gentle examination. The other practical method of assessment of deep wounds is a gloved finger (Cooper, 1990). Both of these techniques are subject to a degree of accuracy dependent upon where the measurement is taken, as this needs to be repeated on reassessment.

Photography

Over the last few years photography has become a popular method of recording wound progress. One reason is that good quality pictures are particularly useful in the light of increasing legal cases. Photographs also provide a detailed picture of the wound. Photography provides a permanent record and successive pictures can be compared for the purpose of detecting improvement or deterioration of the wound (Anthony, 1987).

Louis (1992) suggested that:

Word description and observation of wounds does not provide a complete overall picture. However, a photograph taken correctly can say it all.

Another advantage of using photographs for patient care is that the effects of treatment can be monitored closely and clinicians do not have to have the dressing removed unnecessarily. It is prudent to take not only a photograph of the wound but also measurements of the wound and to record progress on assessment charts. This additional material can then be included in the patient's documentation.

The distance from which a photograph is taken is very important to prevent inaccurate comparisons due to altered visual perceptions. A consistent angle also adds to the accuracy of the wound being photographed (Louis, 1992). Patients may also be motivated by improvements seen in a set of photographs from week to week. This can act as positive reinforcement and help the patient to motivate him/herself to participate in the plan of care.

A photograph of a patient's wound provides an unambiguous image for clinical reimbursement and legal purposes. This is particularly pertinent in the USA as more litigation takes place there.

A patient's photograph, taken on admission, showing damaged skin integrity is evidence that will be of use when investigating a complaint; it will also help settle any doubt in the documentation. It is therefore advisable that photographs are taken on admission if the patient's skin is compromised by any damage clearly caused before admission. Photographs can be used not only for documenting wound history within all healthcare settings, but also for the education of patients, families and other healthcare professionals.

For the best results, medical photographers should be used, as they are trained to take consistent photographs, which allow comparisons between photographic images over a period of time (Melhuish, 1997). A professional photographer will consider whether the detail can be clearly seen and if the wound will be in the centre of the picture with good background and lighting. An autofocus camera is not the ideal, but it is better than no documentation at all and is relatively inexpensive to purchase.

The Polaroid camera is portable and has the facility to provide a set distance of ten inches from which the photograph is taken, making evaluation effortless. The advantage of this method is that the photograph is instantly produced with a grid; however, reprints cannot be made easily. When taking photographs, for whatever reason, the patient's written consent must always be obtained, particularly if the photographs will be used for slides or in published material at a later date. Flanagan (1997) states that if you chose to take your own photographs, some common rules need to be followed (*Table 10.3*)

Table 10.3: Rules for photography
Patient identity should always be kept confidential
Close up shots of the wound need to be in focus to provide good quality photography
The background needs to be green to provide a contrast
Subsequent photographs need to be taken in the same position
Photographs need to be stored in a secure place

Adapted from Flanagan, 1997

Conclusion

Nurses play a crucial role in wound management and need to have a sound knowledge of wound physiology, and the skills to assess the stages of wound healing for accurate documentation. The form of documentation is not important; it can be hand written or computer generated. The use of clear terminology is most important, as is using standardised charts for colour classification and measurement of wounds. This allows easy evaluation by different practitioners. There are numerous methods of measuring wounds; however, some of these are only practical for research purposes and are impractical for everyday use in the ward area.

It appears that the most commonly employed method of measuring a wound is by way of tracing and counting the number of squares on an underlying grid to determine the area. This material can then be placed in the patient's notes. The limitations of each available wound measurement/assessment tool have to be carefully considered.

One of the best forms of documentation is a photograph as it provides a clear and meaningful record of the wound. Photographic documentation may be used in legal cases and, in conjunction with good documentation of nursing notes, can not be misinterpreted. With advancing technology more new techniques will become available in the area of research; however, for everyday use the available techniques need to be simple and quick so as not to interfere unduly with the nurse's increasing workload.

Key points

❖ In the past, nurses have not employed evidence-based nursing practice but have employed anecdotal evidence.

❖ The classification of a wound depends on the knowledge of the practitioner of the physiology of the skin.

❖ For the practitioner to decide if effective wound care is being applied, measurements need to be taken to evaluate the wound's progress.

❖ Photographs also provide a detailed picture of the wound.

References

Ahroni JH, Boyko EJ, Percorarao RE (1993) Reliability of computerised wound surface area determination. *Wounds: A Compendium of Clinical Research and Practice* 4(4): 133–7

Anthony D (1987) The accurate measurement of pressure sores. In: Fielding P, ed. *Research in the Nursing Care of Elderly People*. Wiley and Sons, Chichester: 1–25

Association of Enterostomal Therapists (1987) *Standards of Care for Dermal Wounds*. Association of Enterostomal Therapists, Irvine, California

Bates-Jensen BM, Vredevoe DL, Brecht ML (1992) Validity and reliability of pressure sore status tool. *Decubitus* 5(6): 20–18

Bates-Jensen BM (1995) National pressure ulcer advisory panel proceedings: indices to include in wound healing assessment. *Advances Wound Care* 8(4): 25–8

Benbow M (1995) Parameters of wound assessment. *Br J Nurs* 4(11): 647–51

Bennett G, Moody M (1995) *Wound Care for Health Professionals*. Chapman and Hall, London

Bergstrom N, Bennett MA (1994) *Treatment of Pressure Ulcers. Clinical Practice Guidelines. No. 15. US Department of Health and Human Services*. AHCCR Publications, Rockville, Maryland

Boardman M, Melhuish JM (1994) Hue saturation and intensity in healing wound image. *J Wound Care* 3(7): 314–9

Briggs M, Banks S (1995) *Documenting wound management*. In: Cherry GW, ed. 5th European Conference on Wound Management. Macmillan Magazines, London: 35–6

Brohannan RW, Pfaller BA (1983) Documentation of wound surface area from tracing of wound perimeters. *Phys Therapy* 63(10): 1622–4

Bulstrode CJK, Goode AW (1986) Stereophotogrammetry for measuring rates of cutaneous healing: a comparison with conventional techniques. *Clin Sci* 71: 437–43

Buntinx F, Beckers H (1996) Inter-observer variation in the assessment of skin ulceration. *J Wound Care* **5**(4): 166–70

Collier (1994) Assessing a wound. *Nurs Standard* **8**(49): 3–8

Cooper D (1990) Human wound assessment: status report and implications for clinicians. *Clin Issues Crit Care Nurs* **1**(3): 553–65

Cooper DM (1992) Wound assessment and evaluation of healing. In: Bryant RA, ed. *Acute and Chronic Wound Care: Nursing Management*. Mosby Year Book, St Louis: 69–90

Crisculob GR, Oldfield EH (1988) Measurements of intracranial tissue volume using computed tomographic images and personal computer. *Neurosurgery* **23**: 671–4

Cuzzell JZ (1988) The new RYB colour code. *Am J Nurs* **88**: 1342–6

Dealey C (1994) *The Care of Wounds*. Blackwell Scientific, Oxford

Flanagan M (1992) *Wound Care Society Wound Assessment Leaflet*. Wound Care Society, Northampton

Flanagan M (1996) A practical framework for wound assessment 1: physiology. *Br J Nurs* **5**(22): 1391–7

Flanagan M (1997) Wound healing and management. *Primary Health Care* **7**(4): 31–9

Franz RA, Johnson DA (1992) A compendium of clinical research and practice: stereophotography and computerised image analysis: a three-dimensional method of measuring wound healing. *Wounds* **4**: 58–64

Gentzkow GD (1995) National pressure ulcer advisory panel proceedings: methods for measuring size in pressure ulcers. *Advances Wound Care* **8**(4): 28–45

Gilman TH (1990) Parameters for the measurement of wound closure. *Wounds* **3**: 95–100

Gowland Hopkins NF, Jamieson CW (1983) Antibiotic concentration in the exudate of venous ulcers: prediction of ulcer healing rate. *Br J Surg* **70**: 532–4

Hammersley M, Atkinson P (1991) *Ethnography — Principles in Practice*. Routledge, London

Hampton S (1997) Wound assessment. *Prof Nurse* **12**(12): 55–87

Hansen GL, Sparrow EM, Kokate JY, Leland KJ, Iaizzo PA (1997) Wound status evaluation using colour image processing. *IEEE Transaction Med Imaging* **16**(1): 78–86

Healey F (1995) The reliability and utility of pressure sore grading systems. *J Tiss Viabil* **5**(4): 111–4

Hohn D, Pounce B (1977) Antimicrobial systems of the surgical wound. *Am J Surg* **133**(5): 597–600

Kerstein MD (1997) The scientific basis of healing. *Advances Wound Care* **3**(10): 30–6

Krasner D (1992) The 12 commandments of wound care. *Nursing* **22**(12): 34–42

Kundin JI (1985) Designing and developing a new measuring instrument. *Perioperative Nurse Q* **1**(4): 40–5

Lazarus GS, Cooper DM (1994) Definitions and guidelines for assessment of wounds and evaluation of healing. *Arch Dermatol* **130**: 489–93

Louis DT (1992) Photographing pressure ulcers to enhance documentation. *Decubitus* **5**(4): 44–5

Majeske C (1992) Reliability of wound surface area measures. *Physical Ther* **72**: 138–41

Maklebust J (1995) Pressure ulcer staging systems. *Advances Wound Care* **8**(4): 11–4

Mekkes JR, Westerhof W (1992) A new computer image analysis system designed for evaluating wound debriding products. In: Harding K, ed. *2nd European Conference on Advances in Wound Management*. Macmillian Magazines, London: 4–7

Melhuish JM, Plassman P (1994) Circumference, area and volume of the healing wound. *J Wound Care* **3**(8): 380–4

Melhuish J (1997) Wound care society supplement: know how, a guide to medical photography. *Nurs Times* **93**(7): 64–5

Moody M (1993) Accountability in wound care — a practical approach. *Wound Man* **3**(1): 6–7

Morison MJ (1992) *A Colour Guide to Nursing Management of Wounds*. 1st edn. Wolfe, London

National Pressure Ulcer Advisory Panel (1989) Pressure ulcer prevalence, cost and risk assessment: consensus development conference statement. *Decubitus* **2**(2): 24–8

National Health Service Executive (1993) *Keeping the Record Straight. A Guide for Record Keeping. Nurse and Midwives*. HMSO, London

Palmer RM, Ring EFJ, Legard LA (1989) A digital video technique for radiographs and monitoring ulcers. *J Photog Sci* **37**: 65–7

Plassmann P (1995) Measuring wounds — a guide to the use of wound measurement techniques. *J Wound Care* **4**(6): 269–72

Ramirez AT, Sorof HS, Schwartz MS (1969) Experimental wound healing in man. *Surg Gynae Obstet* **128**: 283–93

Shea JD (1975) Pressure sore classifications and management. *Clin Orth* **112**: 89–100

Taylor RJ (1995) The calculation of linear dimension and image area using a digitising tablet and personal computer. *Int J Clin Monit Comp* **12**: 25–31

Taylor RJ (1997) Mouseyes: an aid to wound measurement using a computer. *J Wound Care* **6**(3): 123–6

Thomas S, Wysocki AE (1990) The healing wound: a comparison of three clinically useful methods of measurement. *Decubitus* **3**(1): 18–25

Torrance C (1983) *Pressure Sores: Aetiology, Treatment and Prevention.* Croom Helm, Beckenham, Kent

United Kingdom Central Council for Nursing, Midwifery and Health Visiting (1992) *Code of Professional Conduct for Nurses, Midwives and Health Visitors.* UKCC, London

United Kingdom Central Council for Nursing, Midwifery and Health Visiting (1997) *Post-registration Education Project.* UKCC, London

United Kingdom Central Council for Nursing, Midwifery and Health Visiting (1998) *Guidelines for Records and Record Keeping.* UKCC, London

Van Rijswijk L, Polansky M (1994) Predictors of time to healing deep pressure ulcers ostomy. *Wound Man* **40**(8): 40–50

Williams E (1997) Assessing the future. *Nurs Times* **93**(23): 76–8

Xakellis GC, Chrischilles EA (1992) Hydrocolloid versus saline-gauze dressings in treating pressure ulcers: a cost-effectiveness analysis. *Arch Phys Med Rehab* **73**: 463–8

Xakellis GC, Frantz RA (1997) NPUAP proceedings, pressure ulcer healing: what is it? what influences it? how is it measured? *Advances Wound Man* **10**(5): 20–6

11

The importance of patients' nutritional status in wound healing

Linda Russell

Good nutritional status is essential for wound healing to take place. Ignoring nutritional status may compromise the patient's ability to heal and subsequently prolong the stages of wound healing. Glucose provides the body with its power source for wound healing and this gives energy for angiogenesis and the deposition of new tissue. Therefore, it is vital that the body receives adequate amounts of glucose to provide additional energy for wound healing. Fatty acids are essential for cell structure and have an important role in the inflammatory process. Wound healing is dependent on good nutrition and the presence of suitable polyunsaturated fatty acids in the diet. Protein deficiency has been demonstrated to contribute to poor healing rates with reduced collagen formation and wound dehiscence. High exudate loss can result in a deficit of as much as 100g of protein in one day. This subsequently needs to be replaced with a high protein diet. Vitamins are also important in wound healing. Vitamin C deficiency contributes to fragile granulation tissue. There is a correlation between low serum albumin and body mass index (BMI) and the development of pressure ulcers. Also, low serum albumin and high Waterlow score have a positive association. The body automatically renews tissue while we are asleep but this does not mean that protein synthesis does not take place during our wakeful hours. Holistic assessment of nutrition and early detection of malnutrition are essential to promote effective wound healing.

Wound healing is an intricate process and is the body's natural response to trauma. When this process is delayed or slowed, problems such as wound infections and keloid scarring are more likely to occur. Patients require adequate levels of protein, vitamins, fats and minerals to support wound healing (Morison *et al*, 1997). A patient with partial- or full-thickness burns or injuries will require a greater calorie intake.

The Panel for the Prediction and Prevention of Pressure Ulcers in Adults (1992) states that patients with pressure ulcers require 30–50 kcal and 1.25–1.50g protein per kg body weight daily. A patient with a grade 3–4 pressure sore requires 2g per day of protein (Chernoff and Milton, 1990). By comparison, the estimated average protein requirements for a 50–55-year-old male are 53g/d, and for a female 46g/d (Department of Health, 1991).

Wound healing is a complex process and nutrition plays a crucial role in the formation of new tissue. It is suggested that:

Alteration in nutritional status or intake preceding or during injury may clearly alter the normal wound healing response.

Pinchcofsky-Devin, 1994

If the body's defences are low, replacement of tissue will be slower. Neglecting the nutritional health of the individual may totally compromise all the wound management undertaken (Wallace, 1994).

The body's response to a wound sustained through trauma, surgery or injury is to increase protein requirements. Initially, there is a fall in the metabolic rate in response to the trauma, but then it will rise again provided enough protein is available from the patient's reserves. As a result, fat and lean body mass will be broken down to provide extra energy. This is known as a catabolic state (Guest and Pearson, 1997). After surgery, additional nutrition will be required for wound healing. It is suggested that:

Best surgical and nursing care available will not heal the wound if there is inadequate nutritional substrate to make new tissue.

Pinchcofsky-Devin, 1994

It is well established that improved nutritional status will improve healing (Holmes *et al*, 1987; Guest and Pearson, 1997). However, a poor nutritional intake is often found in patients who develop pressure ulcers and can result in delayed wound healing. This can result in a continuous cycle if it is not broken.

A patient who is malnourished can be given many forms of energy supplements. One of the most concentrated energy sources is fat, which has twice the amount of calories per gram than carbohydrates, eg. cakes, biscuits and chocolates. The patient may, or may not, find these foodstuffs more desirable than nutritional supplements or drinks (Guest and Pearson, 1997).

Glucose

Glucose provides the body with vital energy. In a wound, the cellular infiltrate of leucocytes and macrophages use glucose for aerobic glycolysis, which provides the energy for the production of factors that stimulate fibroblast production and collagen synthesis (McLaren, 1991). As a result of an injury, the body responds by developing hyperglycaemia, induced by increased glucagon and adrenaline and a reduction in insulin, which increases glycogenolysis in the liver. This is part of the body's survival mechanism to supply it with additional energy.

Depending on the extent of the injury, the need for extra energy varies. Wilmore (1977) demonstrated that wound glucose utilisation reached 175g per day in the case of patients with 42% burns.

Small wounds produce little effect on the metabolism, but extensive injuries such as burns can cause a significant rise in energy expenditure and hence requirements (Meyer *et al*, 1994). The effective production of energy depends on the body's capacity for aerobic metabolism, supported by angiogenesis — new blood vessels of short intercapillary distances, that are formed by the process of angiogenesis (endothelial buds that lay down), form new granulation tissue (Madden, 1983; Morison *et al*, 1997).

Fatty acids

The role of fatty acids in the inflammatory response and tissue formation is becoming increasingly understood. Polyunsaturated fatty acids (PUFAs) are responsible for integrity of cell membrane structure and function. The release of membrane eicosanoids, chemicals involved in the inflammatory response, sends the biochemical message to initiate wound healing.

The metabolism of PUFAs produces prostaglandin E_3 and leukotrienes, which have vasodilatory and anti-inflammatory actions. The ω-6 PUFA metabolites include prostaglandins E_2 and I_2, which help mediate the inflammatory response, platelet aggregation and vasoconstriction (McLaren, 1991; Morison *et al*, 1997). Immunocompetent cells can synthesise eicosanoids from PUFAs, but this depends on the availability of ω-6 PUFA in the cellular pool. In turn, this activity is dependent on the nutritional intake, and this affects the phospholipase activity (Morison *et al*, 1997).

The ω series of polyunsaturated fatty acids, eg. eicosapentaenoic (20:5ω-3) and docosahexaenoic (22:6ω-3) can be found in fish oils (Edwards *et al*, 1995). Increasing ω-3 PUFAs' dietary manipulation could result in reduced incorporation of ω-6 PUFA, thus reducing prostaglandin E_2 (PGE$_2$) production and resulting in altered T cells proliferative response, which could potentially benefit wounds that are in a persistent state of clinical inflammation caused by overactive macrophages (Cerra, 1991). This may occur where there is persistent inflammation, partly caused by the overactivity of macrophages (McLaren, 1991).

Gottslich *et al* (1990) demonstrated that an enteral feeding formula containing ω-3 fatty acids reduces the incidence of wound infection after burns.

Further research is required to determine the therapeutic dose of PUFA that is required to optimise effective healing in all types of wounds (Morison *et al*, 1997).

Protein

A high protein diet is advantageous in the healing of pressure ulcers in long-stay elderly patients (Breslow and Bergstrom, 1994).

Protein requirements for an acutely ill patient are 1.5–2.5kg in order to avoid negative nitrogen balance, which would place the patient in a state of anabolism (Chernoff and Milton, 1990). However, this may not necessarily happen in patients who are critically ill. Patients given high protein diets may require a high fluid intake to prevent renal failure (Pinchcofsky-Devin, 1994).

Protein deficiency contributes to poor wound healing by prolonging the inflammatory process, impairing collagen synthesis, and increasing the risk of wound dehiscence. A further problem encountered is secondary oedema due to hypoalbuminaemia — low protein levels for a very long period of time, which can be a long-term sequel to protein malnutrition (Morton, 1995).

Wound healing requires a large amount of energy because of the synthesis of the components needed for tissue repair. All the nutrients are transported around the body in the blood supply, which has to be adequately oxygenated. Many elderly patients have an underlying pathology, such as poor blood supply and reduced oxygen carriage, owing to their age. Wounds that are compromised by poor blood supply heal slower than well perfused wounds.

Albumin provides a source of amino acids for a healing wound. Cells can acquire albumin from the intravascular and extravascular compartments because albumin is freely permeable across cell membranes. At the site of injury, permeability may be increased, thus increasing plasma protein availability which appears to facilitate wound healing (Powanda and Moyer, 1981). Copious wound exudate can use as much as 100g of protein per day (Thomas, 1994). Therefore, the patient's diet will need to compensate for this loss.

Oxygen expenditure of the body is increased during sleep and causes catabolism (Shapiro *et al*, 1993). Tissue renewal also takes place while we are asleep (Adam and Oswald, 1983). Growth hormone is released during sleep, aiding wound healing, as well as resting the patient's body (Adam and Oswald, 1983). Protein synthesis also occurs during the wakeful hours, and this enables the restoration of body tissue, but plenty of sleep and rest are necessary to promote wound healing.

Vitamins

Alvarez and Gilbreath (1982) suggest that vitamins play a vital role in wound healing. Vitamin supplements may need to be increased by 10–20 times the normal recommended dose. The reason for this increase is the amount excreted by the body, reduced absorption and drug interaction, as well as their utilisation in the increased metabolic process during wound healing.

Vitamin C

Vitamin C is vital for collagen synthesis. However, the role of vitamin C is not fully understood: '... only that it is a stimulant for fibroblast cell division and subsequently collagen synthesis' (Pinchcofsky-Devin, 1994).

In vitro studies have demonstrated increased uptake of vitamin C during phagocytosis (Shilotry, 1977; Leibowitz and Seigal, 1978). Vitamin C may increase the activity of leucocytes and macrophages to the wound. *In vitro* studies also showed that ascorbic acid may increase the activation of leucocytes and macrophages at, and attraction to, the injury site (Shilotry, 1977; Leibowitz and Seigal, 1978).

Goode and Burns (1992) demonstrated a connection between low concentrations of leucocytes, vitamin C and pressure ulcers in patients with fractured neck or femur injuries. Vitamin C supplementation has demonstrated that more rapid healing of pressure ulcers took place (Taylor *et al*, 1994). An explanation for this may be that the patients were in a deficient state. However, there has been little research into this apparent relationship, probably because of difficulties in measuring the levels of vitamin C.

Those patients at risk of pressure ulcers and who were poor eaters had an intake of significantly less vitamin C than patients who did not sustain pressure ulcers (Bergstrom and Braden, 1992). Vitamin C deficiency causes prolonged wound healing because of increased capillary fragility (Irvin and Challopadhyay, 1978).

Vitamin C deficiency increases the risk of wound dehiscence and contributes to fragile granulation tissue. Vitamin C is another vital co-factor for enzymes concerned with collagen synthesis (Casey, 1998). Open wounds require a great deal more collagen and new capillary growth. This process is dependent on the patient's nutritional status being favourable in order to produce healthy granulation tissue (Flanagan, 1998).

Vitamin A

Vitamin A stimulates differentiation in fibroblasts and collagen synthesis, thereby quickening the healing process and increasing tensile strength (Pinchcofsky-Devin, 1994). Another function of vitamin A is a humoral defence mechanism to help fight wound infections locally or systemically. Vitamin A compensates for the catabolic effect that glucocorticosteroids exert on wound healing (Ehrlich and Hunt, 1968).

Greenwald (1990) demonstrated that vitamin A enhances the healing of tendons. Vitamin A used topically can enhance epithelialisation (Smith *et al*, 1986).

Vitamin E

Vitamin E facilitates wound healing by enhancing the immune response. However, the role of this vitamin in wound healing is controversial as some reviews state it is harmful *in vitro* on tendon healing (Greenwald, 1990), while others say it is beneficial (Morton, 1995).

Vitamin E prevents lipid peroxidation of PUFAs in cell membranes by oxygen free radicals, thereby assisting anti-oxidant defence and wound healing (McLaren, 1991).

Decreased levels of vitamin E are associated with shortened lifespans of red and white blood cells (Pinchcofsky-Devin, 1994). A daily dose of vitamin E should not exceed 67mg, as a higher dose can cause fibrosis, which subsequently delays wound healing (Taylor and Goodinson-McLaren, 1992).

Vitamin K

Vitamin K is known for its role in haemostatic clot formation over the injury site.

It is a prerequisite for wound healing (Pinchcofsky-Devin, 1994).

Vitamin B complex

Several vitamins form the Vitamin B complex: thiamine/riboflavin, pyridoxine, folic acid and pantothenate (Chernoff, 1996). They have various roles:

- assisting leucocytes and antibody formation
- intermediary roles in metabolism
- assisting essential co-factors in enzyme activity.

Thiamine/riboflavin and pyridoxine are important in the formation of collagen matrix (Alvarez and Gilbreath, 1982).

Vitamin B_6 assayed by high performance liquid chromatography (HPLC) has been demonstrated to be statistically lower in patients who fracture their hip in low impact falls than in patients whose hip fractures had elective surgery (Reynolds and Baine, 1992), suggesting that further research into interaction of these two vitamins may be needed.

Trace elements

It is well documented that trace elements, such as zinc, copper and iron, play an important role in wound healing, as many are co-factors for enzymes involved in the process of new tissue formation (Morison *et al*, 1997). There is no overall factor that underpins the effects of wound healing, and further research is still needed as to the key micronutrients involved. It is stated that:

Zinc status does not appear to be a significant factor in the development of pressure sores.

Lewis, 1996

However, zinc therapy has also been demonstrated to be of benefit in patients with poorly healing surgical wounds (Henzel and DeWeese, 1970). Currently, there are insufficient studies to draw any conclusions as to the role of zinc in the healing of pressure ulcers.

Iron is necessary for the formation of collagen and transportation of oxygen to the tissues. Copper is required for the collagen matrix. An important fact is that erythrocyte production requires both copper and iron (Pinchcofsky-Devin, 1994). Guest and Pearson (1997) have shown that copper increases tensile strength of collagen.

To optimise wound healing, sufficient protein, energy, vitamin and mineral requirements have to be available or else corrected by nutritional supplementation. It is suggested that:

Nutrition assumes an equal footing with other time honoured pathogenic considerations in wound prevention and treatment.

Pinchcofsky-Devin, 1994

Serum albumin

Serum albumin values represent the body's albumin production and breakdown balance. A certain amount of extracellular albumin is stored in the skin and the rest in the muscles and viscera. Low serum albumin level results from decreased synthesis, increased catabolism and excessive loss into tissues. Most cases of decreased serum albumin are caused by protein malnutrition. When a patient has inadequate calorie intake but lacks protein in the diet, adult Kwashiorkor-like malnutrition may occur (Pinchcofsky-Devin, 1994).

A connection between serum albumin and the formation of pressure ulcers has not been shown (Bergstrom and Braden, 1992).

Strauss and Margolis (1996) have stated that:

Recognizing deficits in the indices before they reach values that may reflect and jeopardize healing may help minimize morbidity and mortality in the population.

Anthony *et al* (2000) carried out a prospective study of 773 patients over the age of sixty-four years with a hospital stay of at least one week. Using the Hospital Information Support System to explain the data, patients' Waterlow scores, serum albumin levels, and sodium levels were analysed using SPSS for logistic regression and discriminate analysis. A ROC (receiver operating characteristics) curve was used for sensitivity and specificity of the Waterlow scores at various thresholds. It was statistically demonstrated that high Waterlow scores and low serum albumin were strongly correlated ($P<0.001$) for patients who developed pressure ulcers. This study recommends that serum albumin can be assessed to give a better predictive power to the Waterlow score and can also provide greater sensitivity to identify patients who will develop a pressure ulcer.

Body mass index

Rudman and Feller (1987) demonstrated the relationship between an annual death rate and percentage of ideal body weight (IBW). Patients with actual body weight >100% of IBW had an annual death rate of 9.8%, compared with an annual death rate of 26.3% for those patients with an actual body weight of <80% of IBW. An IBW of <85% has been associated with numerous problems related to malnutrition (Harvey *et al*, 1981).

The surface area of a pressure ulcer is inversely related to the body mass index (Breslow, 1991). The importance of oral supplementation is that when used correctly it can improve wound healing and avoid the need for enteral feeding (Himes, 1997).

The IBW and serum albumin should form a part of the clinical assessment of pressure ulcers (Strauss and Margolis, 1996). This information gives an overall profile of the patient's condition and the severity of a pressure ulcer. Early nutritional assessment of these patients is vital, as recommended by the

British Association for Parenteral and Enteral Nutrition (1994). Early treatment to rectify nutritional deficits will promote healing and reduce morbidity and mortality rates, particularly in elderly people.

Conclusion

The literature reveals that wound healing is very complex and correct amounts of proteins, energy, vitamins, minerals and a good blood supply are essential for the formation of collagen, allowing nutrients and energy to be carried to the wound.

More research is required as to the importance of nutritional status in patients with pressure ulcers, and also the role which proteins, vitamins and micronutrients play and the quantities of each required for healing. It appears that these roles are not fully understood.

Serum albumin is a recognised surrogate biochemical marker, offering an indication of the patient's nutritional status, but it does not provide the answer to the patient's risk of developing pressure ulcers. Serum albumin used alongside the Waterlow score will help to highlight patients who have a high risk of developing pressure ulcers (Anthony *et al*, 2000).

Nutrition supplementation and pressure area care will prevent unnecessary suffering from pressure ulcers. Continuous assessment of a patient's nutritional status is very important, with reassessment carried out weekly or when the condition changes (Rollins, 1997).

The nurse is the ideal person to make assessment of a patient's wound healing and then decide on appropriate nutrition, either by food or artificial means.

Key Points

❖ Patients require adequate levels of calories, protein, vitamins and minerals to support wound healing.

❖ Alteration in nutritional status, intake preceeding or during injury may clearly alter the normal wound healing response.

❖ Depending on the extent of the injury, the need for extra energy varies.

❖ Polyunsaturated fatty acids are responsible for integrity of the cell membrane structure and function.

References

Adam K, Oswald I (1983) Protein synthesis, bodily renewal and the sleep–wake cycle. *Clin Sci* **62**(6): 561–7

Alvarez OM, Gilbreath R (1982) Thiamine influences on colagen during the granulation of ski wounds. *J Surg Res* **32**: 24–31

Anthony D, Reynolds T, Russell LJ (2000) An investigation into the use of serum albumin in pressure sore prediction. *J Adv Nurs* **32**(2): 359–65

Bergstrom N, Braden B (1992) A prospective study of pressure sore risk among institutionalized elderly. *J Am Geriatr Soc* **40**: 747–58

Breslow R (1991) Nutritional status and dietary intake of patients with pressure ulcers: review of research literature 1943–1989. *Decubitus* **4**(1): 16–21

Breslow R, Bergstrom N (1994) Nutrition prediction of ulcers. *J Am Diet Assoc* **94**(11): 1301–4

British Association for Parenteral and Enteral Nutrition (1994) *Organization of Nutritional Support in Hospitals*. ADM and C, Biddenden, Kent

Casey G (1998) The importance of nutrition in wound healing. *Nurs Standard* **13**(3 Suppl): 51–6

Cerra FB (1991) Nutrient modulation of inflammatory and immune function. *Am J Surg* **161**: 202–34

Chernoff R (1996) Policy: nutrition standards for treatment of pressure ulcers. *Nutrition Reviews* **54**(1): 43–4

Chernoff R, Milton K (1990) The effect of high protein liquid formulas (replete) on decubitus ulcer healing in the long-term tube-fed institutionalized patients. *J Am Diet Assoc* **90**(9): A–130 (abstract)

DoH (1991) *Dietary Reference Values for Food and Energy and Nutrients for the UK*. Department of Health, London

Edwards CRW, Bouchier IAD, Haslett C *et al* (1995) *Davidson's Principles and Practice of Medicine*. 17th edn. Churchill Livingstone, London: 551–3

Ehrlich HP, Hunt TK (1968) Effect of cortisone and vitamin A on wound healing. *Ann Surg* **167**: 324–8

Flanagan M (1998) The characteristics and formation of granulation tissue. *J Wound Care* **7**(10): 508–10

Goode HF, Burns E (1992) Vitamin C depletion and pressure sores in elderly patients with femoral neck fractures. *Br Med J* **305**: 925–7

Gottslich MM, Jenkins M, Warden GD *et al* (1990) Differential effects of three dietary regimens on selected outcomes: variables in burn patients. *J Parenter Enter Nutr* **14**(3): 225–34

Greenwald D (1990) Intrinsic tendon, healing *in vitro*: biomechanical analysis and effects of vitamins A and E. *Curr Surg* **47**: 440–3

Guest C, Pearson D (1997) Wound care — recovery on a plate. *Nurs Times* **93**(46): 84–6

Harvey KN, Moldawer LL, Bistrian BR *et al* (1981) Biologic measures for the formulation of a hospital prognostic index. *Am J Clin Nutr* **34**: 2013–22

Henzel JH, DeWeese MS (1970) Zinc concentration within healing wounds: significance of postoperative zincuria on availability and requirements during tissue repair. *Arch Surg* **100**: 349–57

Himes D (1997) Nutritional supplements in the treatment of pressure ulcers: practical perspectives. *Adv Wound Care* **10**(1): 30

Holmes R, Macchiano K, Jhangiani SS (1987) Combating pressure sores nutritionally. *Am J Nurs* **87**(10): 1301–3

Irvin TT, Challopadhyay DK (1978) Ascorbic acid requirements in postoperative patients. *Am J Surg* **147**: 49

Leibowitz B, Seigal BV (1978) Ascorbic acid neutrophil function and immune response. *Int J Vitam Nutr Res* **48**: 159–64

Lewis B (1996) Zinc and vitamin C in the aetiology of pressure sores. *J Wound Care* **5**(10): 483–4

McLaren S (1991) Nutrition and wound healing. In: Harding K, ed. *1st European Conference on Advances in Wound Management*. Macmillan Magazine, London: 67–78

Madden J (1983) Wound healing and wound care. In: Dudnick SJ, ed. *Manual of Preoperative and Postoperative Care*. WB Saunders, Philadelphia: 170–2

Meyer NA, Muller MJ, Herndon DN (1994) Nutrient support of healing wound. *New Horiz* **2**(2): 202–14

Morison M, Moffatt C, Briden-Nixon J et al (1997) In: Morison M, ed. *Nursing Management of Chronic Wounds*. 2nd edn. Mosby, London: 27–51

Morton K (1995) Nutrition and wound care. In: Cherry GW, ed. *Proceedings of the 5th European Conference on Advances in Wound Management*. Macmillan Magazines, London: 31–4

Panel for the Prediction and Prevention of Pressure Ulcers in Adults (1992) *Pressure Ulcers in Adults: Prediction and Prevention*. Agency for Health Care Policy and Research, Public Health Service, US Department of Health and Human Services, Clinical Practice Guidelines, 92-0047, Rockville, Maryland

Pinchcofsky-Devin G (1994) Nutrition and wound healing. *J Wound Care* **3**(5): 231–4

Powanda MC, Moyer ED (1981) Plasma proteins and wound healing. *Surg Gynecol Obstet* **153**: 857

Reynolds, Baine T (1992) A simple internally standardized isocractic HPLC assay for vitamin B6 in human serum. *Liquid Chromatography* **15**: 897–914

Rollins H (1997) Nutrition and wound healing. *Nurs Standard* **11**(51): 49–52

Rudman D, Feller AG (1987) Relation of serum albumin concentration to death rate in nursing home men. *J Parent Enter Nutr* **11**(4): 360–3

Shapiro C, Devins GM, Hussian MRG (1993) Sleep problems in patients with medical illness. *Br Med J* **306**: 1532–5

Shilotry PG (1977) Phagocytosis and leucocyte enzymes in ascorbic acid-deficient guinea pigs. *J Nutr* **107**: 1507–12

Smith K, Zarbiokas L, Ditlake R (1986) Cortisone, vitamin A and wound healing. *J Surg Res* **40**: 120

Strauss EA, Margolis DJ (1996) Malnutrition in patients with pressure ulcers: morbidity, mortality, and clinically practical assessments. *Adv Wound Care* **9**(5): 37–40

Taylor S, Goodinson-McLaren S (1992) *Special Nutritional Requirements and Uses of Enteral and Parenteral Nutrition. Nutritional Support: A Team Approach.* Wolfe, London

Taylor TV, Rimmer S, Day B *et al* (1994) Ascorbic acid supplementation in the treatment of pressure sores. *Lancet* **ii**: 544

Thomas B, ed (1994) Catabolic states. In: *British Dietetic Association. Manual of Dietetic Practice.* Blackwell Scientific, Oxford: 537–49

Wallace E (1994) Feeding the wound: nutrition and wound care. *Br J Nurs* **3**(13): 662–7

Wilmore DW (1977) Influence of burn wound on local and systemic responses to injury. *Ann Surg* **186**: 444–58

Nursing aspects of pressure ulcer prevention and therapy

Fiona Culley

Pressure ulcers remain a significant problem in hospitals and domestic settings, affecting people of all ages, social class and race. Associated complications may be life threatening, eg. sepsis and osteomyelitis. Other less dangerous, but nevertheless compromising outcomes such as pain, discomfort and low self-esteem and body image can cause personal suffering, and may add extra demand upon limited resources. The exact state of pressure ulcer occurrence remains difficult to determine, particularly in the community. Recent trends in pressure area management emphasise a multidisciplinary approach, eroding traditional perceptions of pressure ulcers as solely a nursing problem. Written from a nursing perspective, this chapter summarises principles of good practice relating to pressure ulcer prevention and therapy, emphasising the importance of documenting observed events, rather than assumptions or opinions, and the need for healthcare professionals to approach problems and needs from a collaborative stance. Pressure ulcer risk assessment and classification are discussed, and an overview of nutrition, repositioning, selecting support surfaces, principles of wound management, and skin care are considered.

The exact state of pressure ulcer occurrence in the UK remains difficult to determine, particularly in community settings. Dissemination of prevalence and incidence rates, a growth in the number of tissue viability specialist posts and minimising risk as part of the clinical governance agenda are some of the factors raising the profile of pressure ulcer prevention and management strategies. Subsequently, the Department of Health commissioned the Royal College of Nursing to develop clinical guidelines on pressure ulcer risk assessment and prevention. These have since been inherited and disseminated by the National Institute for Clinical Excellence (2001) whose function as a special health authority is to promote clinical effectiveness. The Department of Health (2001) have also included pressure ulcers as one of eight distinct categories of patient focused benchmarks — aimed at encouraging clinicians to review their own practice against set criteria and discuss practical solutions to achieving best practice. A number of common issues are addressed in the above such as risk assessment, repositioning and skin care. Educational initiatives, risk reporting, audit and research programmes are necessary to support application of the above, and are critical constituents of quality improvement and accountable practice. Healthcare providers are continuing to forge links with academic institutions to this end.

At a more extensive level the National Pressure Ulcer Advisory Panel (NPUAP) was established in the USA in 1989 to provide a forum for expert opinion, to guide research, education and public policy. Members of the panel who include representatives from the healthcare professions, as well as equipment manufacturers, have produced comprehensive clinical practice guidelines, based upon scientific evidence and clinical expertise (Agency for Health Care Policy and Research [AHCPR], 1994). A similar approach has been adopted by the European Pressure Ulcer Advisory Panel (EPUAP), gathering experts from fourteen European countries and producing guidelines (EPUAP, 1998a, b) with the aim of improving pressure ulcer prevention and therapy.

Risk assessment

While many examples of good practice have been reported in the literature, and shared at conferences as well as through professional interest groups such as the Tissue Viability Society, Wound Care Society and United Wound Management Education Forum, examples of fragmented approaches to pressure area management have been observed in clinical settings. The National Audit Commission (1995) highlighted some serious lapses in pressure sore prevention in the elderly which were mainly due to poor risk assessment and inadequate documentation and communication of care. O'Dea (1993) revealed that 33% of hospital patients with identified pressure damage remained nursed on standard hospital mattresses. During the same period it was estimated that pressure sores were costing the NHS £320m in prolonged hospital stays. The true costs of pressure sores remain impossible to quantify, although a clearer picture of some expenditure, such as equipment funding and litigation costs, is beginning to emerge.

Tingle (1997) cites a number of clinical negligence cases that have resulted in claims for compensation against acute NHS Trusts and independent nursing homes as a result of pressure damage. A more recent example is that of *Stacey v Sheffield University Hospital NHS Trust 2000*. The Health Service Commissioner (Ombudsman) (Health Service Commissioner 2000 and 2001) also reports on a number of cases attributed to failures in pressure ulcer risk assessment and review. Examples include one Trust reported to have sent a patient home 'with no dressings for a pressure ulcer', while a second 'failed to assess the patient's vulnerability to pressure ulcers frequently enough'.

The obligation of professional accountability for acts and omissions relating to the duty of care is explicitly communicated to nurses via the UKCC's *Code of Professional Conduct* (UKCC, 1992a). Pressure ulcer risk assessment is part of being accountable, and the measurement of commonly recognised intrinsic and extrinsic risk factors may help to support decision making. Risk factors must be documented (UKCC, 1998) and, more importantly, reviewed and acted upon.

Like other aspects of care, assessment, reassessment and evaluation of the patient's pressure sore risk status are the responsibility of the registered nurse with the relevant knowledge and comprehension of the complex aetiology of pressure sores. The UKCC (1992a, b) specifies that registered nurses, healthcare assistants and student nurses must not work beyond their level of competence. Effective risk management is dependent on an appropriate skill mix, for which the employing organisation is answerable.

In many healthcare contexts, formally established pressure ulcer risk assessment scales such as Norton (Norton *et al*, 1962), Waterlow (1985) and Braden (Bergstrom and Braden, 1987) are used to encourage systematic evaluation of an individual's at-risk status. Although such tools have been criticised for their lack of validity and reliability and weak predictive value (Bridel, 1993), they remain a useful aide-memoire to prompt review of the commonly recognised causative factors of tissue damage. They are not intended to prescribe specific pressure reducing or relieving support surfaces, but rather to indicate the degree of risk, and the risk factors that particularly relate to an individual's condition at any given time.

If the employing authority does not use an established assessment tool, it should be able to demonstrate how patients/clients are assessed as being at risk, by whom and when. Undoubtedly, other members of the multidisciplinary healthcare team may significantly contribute to risk assessment and management, and a collaborative approach is a critical success factor.

The patient's management is communicated through accurate documentation, which may at some time be needed as reference for investigation of complaints, or even be subpoenaed by a court of law as documentary evidence. In addition to written notes, photographic records can prove invaluable. Where possible, photographs should be taken by a trained medical photographer. Increasing use of electronic data in tissue viability practice has been reported upon (Newton *et al*, 2000). In such cases ethical and legal principles which govern other types of record keeping should be adhered to as well as Health Service Circular 1998/153. Principles of consent and confidentiality should always be honoured. As part of assessment, there should be a record of the degree of skin and tissue damage. Classification (grading) of such information is of prime importance in facilitating communication between staff, to help monitor healing.

Classification (grading) of pressure ulcers

Although several methods exist for classifying or grading pressure ulcers (David *et al*, 1983; Torrance, 1983; Reid and Morison, 1994; EPUAP, 1998b), they all use the same approach, ie. allocating a score to the skin structures and other tissues involved. Like risk assessment, classification is dependent upon an understanding of the related anatomy, and is the responsibility of a suitably experienced registered nurse.

Classification can be particularly difficult in darkly pigmented skin, as blanching or non-blanching hyperaemia and superficial epidermal breaks can be very hard to detect. Similarly, necrotic pressure ulcers are difficult to classify as the full extent of tissue damage cannot be seen until the area is debrided. Also, most classification systems make no provision for the appearance of blistered skin.

While it is sometimes complicated, pressure ulcer classification should not be abandoned, but needs to be an integral part of nursing documentation, so that a clear account of when tissue damage was first identified and the outcomes of care are evident. Once risk assessment and classification have been carried out, the necessary principles of pressure ulcer prevention and therapy can be applied.

Principles of good practice

Skin care

The maintenance of a good skin condition can greatly minimise the risk of tissue breakdown. Healthy skin will be clean and well hydrated. Skin over bony prominences should not be massaged or rubbed, as this will exacerbate friction and could cause tissue damage (Dyson, 1978; Ek *et al*, 1985). An increase in humidity and moisture exacerbates skin maceration, compromising tissue viability; consequently, plastic sheeting and layers of incontinence padding, for example, should be avoided wherever possible, or at least be changed at the earliest opportunity. Placing extra layers between the skin and the support surface is likely to reduce its effectiveness.

Mechanical skin injury from friction may be reduced by the careful application of barrier dressings such as film dressings (Hall, 1983; Hampton, 1998); however, if film dressings are used, care must be taken to ensure that they stay in place, and do not wrinkle, as this can cause additional risk to tissues.

Nutrition

Patients with complex wounds are at greater risk of malnutrition because of increased metabolic demands, increased loss of nutrients and poor dietary intake due to loss of interest and appetite. People with pressure ulcers that produce copious amounts of exudate are at particular risk. The British Association of Parenteral and Enteral Nutrition (BAPEN, 1994) advocates that all patients at risk of, or diagnosed as being malnourished, should undergo nutritional assessment on, or before, admission to hospital, and have access to a multi-disciplinary nutritional support team. In reality, however, many healthcare providers may not have the resources to meet this objective. A report by Maryon-Davis and Bristow (1999) revealed that 40% of patient meals in hospital were uneaten or thrown in the bin, costing an approximate £144m. In addition, the escalating costs of tissue breakdown or delayed healing as a result of malnutrition may go unrecognised.

Repositioning

For most patients, regular repositioning is an effective strategy towards reducing and/or relieving interface pressure — the amount of pressure generated between the patient's skin and the support surface (Fletcher, 1996). Of primary importance is the patient's mobility. Friction and shear may occur when the patient is moving in bed, or from bed to chair (Dealey, 1997). The Manual Handling Operations Regulations (Health and Safety Executive, 1992) have helped to improve awareness and technique, as well as increased access to a variety of mechanical aids. Appropriate training in the use of such aids is imperative, as misuse can also cause tissue damage.

A repositioning schedule should be agreed, recorded and established for each person 'at risk' (NICE, 2001). It remains unclear how often a person should be moved, and even when pressure relieving/reducing support surfaces are used, regular repositioning remains important for promoting comfort and assisting with pulmonary drainage. It is recommended that those considered to be acutely at risk of developing pressure ulcers should restrict chair sitting to less than two hours until their general condition improves (NICE, 2001; EPUAP, 1998a).

An alternative to traditional positioning techniques is the use of the 30° tilt. With this technique, a pillow is used to tilt the patient at an angle of 30° when lying in bed. This has been shown to reduce interface pressure on the buttocks (Preston, 1988). However, it is not suitable for all patients. For instance, those with contractures or muscle spasm may have difficulty in tolerating the position, or may be unable to straighten their limbs sufficiently (Dealey, 1997).

Using pressure relieving/reducing support surfaces

As part of a wider treatment plan, another major aspect of pressure ulcer prevention and therapy in hospitals and domestic settings is the use of pressure ulcer prevention devices. Clark and Fletcher (1999) report more than 200 pressure relieving/reducing systems to choose from, undoubtedly causing confusion in practice. Despite the availability of a wide range of equipment, for both rental and purchase, there is little evidence to support the efficacy of some devices (Hitch, 1995; Fletcher, 1996) and no compelling evidence that one support surface consistently performs better than all others under all circumstances (AHCPR, 1994). While capillary closing pressure is a measure of the effectiveness of support systems, its measurement is impractical and unlikely to be performed within the care environment. However, evidence of non-blanching hyperaemia should be regarded as a reliable clinical indicator that the existing support surface is not adequately relieving localised pressure, and an explanation of how care and equipment use was modified should be documented. Within the UK, the number of field-based clinical trials appears to be increasing, with manufacturing companies working in collaboration with hospital personnel, primary health staff, and academic institutions.

Dealey (1997) reports on a national political debate, which highlighted *The Health of the Nation* (Department of Health, 1991) targets and indicated a need for a specialist nurse knowledgeable in the use of pressure-relieving equipment, to reduce the complexity of product selection and usage. Several factors influence the selection of equipment (*Table 12.1*). Equal attention should be paid to the patient's need for support surfaces when seated as well as in bed.

Wound management

Once tissue damage is identified and classified, it is necessary to select appropriate topical therapy based upon holistic wound assessment, taking into account the multiplicity of factors known to promote healing. The management of patients with wounds is a complex activity, encompassing more than simply the selection of an appropriate dressing product.

Recent advances in the development of wound contact materials, however, have resulted in a rapid proliferation of different types of dressings, making the selection of an appropriate product confusing. An established framework offering criteria for the optimum wound dressing is that of Turner (1982) shown in *Table 12.2*.

Commonly used contemporary wound dressings in the UK include alginates, enzymes, foams, hydrocolloids, hydrogels and film membranes. Local and systemic infection must be reduced with appropriate antibiotic therapy. Most modern dressings are reported to be comfortable to wear, with dressing changes generally less painful than those associated with traditional applications. Some difficulties in obtaining the complete range of dressings are reported by practitioners, particularly those involved in community care where drug tariffs have restricted the range of dressings available.

On rarer occasions, chronic pressure ulcers may require surgical intervention, most commonly skin grafts and tissue flaps (Black and Black, 1987). Where such surgery is indicated the patient is referred to the specialist plastic surgeon, following a comprehensive health assessment.

Table 12.1: Factors influencing the selection of equipment
Resources
Risk status
Condition and comfort of the patient
Patient's weight and build
Acceptability to the patient (or resident) and carer
Degree of tissue damage
Ability to tolerate a moving, rather than non-moving surface
Safety factors

Source: Young, 1992

Table 12.2: Criteria of an ideal dressing
Removes excess exudate and toxic components
Maintains high humidity at wound-dressing interface
Allows gaseous exchange
Provides thermal insulation
Impermeable to micro-organisms
Free from particulate and toxic contaminants
Removable without causing trauma

Source: Turner, 1982

Conclusion

As more is understood about the complex nature of pressure ulcer prevention and management, the relationship between social and political influences and health care becomes increasingly apparent. With appropriate education, reflection and clinical evidence, it is hoped that practitioners will respond positively to the many challenges of pressure ulcer prevention and therapy, and contribute towards the development of standards of good practice. Although a lack of consensus may appear to impair the development of risk assessment and classification tools, it is anticipated that established forums such as EPUAP, Tissue Viability Society, Wound Care Society, the National Institute for Clinical Excellence and the Royal College of Nursing will promote further dialogue and action. Keeping pressure ulcers on the wider political agenda should heighten awareness of the extent of the problem, and prompt regular appraisal of professional boundaries.

Effective pressure ulcer prevention and therapy strategies rely upon many different areas of expertise, encompassing physiological, psychosocial, legal and ethical, and financial perspectives. Each of these areas needs to be examined through further qualitative and quantitative studies, if pressure area management is to be appropriately resourced and developed.

Key points

❖ Dissemination of prevalence and incidence data, the clinical governance agenda, and a growth in the tissue viability nurse population, are among the influences raising the profile of pressure ulcer strategies within healthcare organisations.

❖ Fragmented approaches to pressure area management continue and may be reduced by education initiatives and research programmes aimed at supporting the development of best practice.

❖ The evidence underpinning tissue viability practice should encompass physiological, psychosocial, legal and ethical and financial issues, each being interdependent.

❖ The escalating costs of tissue breakdown and delayed healing are impossible to quantify, and often go unrecognised.

❖ Assessment, reassessment and evaluation of pressure sore risk status are the responsibility of registered nurses with the related knowledge and understanding of the complex aetiology of pressure ulcer development.

References

Agency for Health Care Policy and Research (1994) *Treatment of Pressure Ulcers, Clinical Practice Guideline No 15.* United States Department of Health and Human Services, Rockville, USA

British Association of Parenteral and Enteral Nutrition (1994) *Standards and Guidelines for Nutritional Support for Patients and Hospitals.* BAPEN, Maidenhead

Bergstrom N, Braden B (1987) The Braden scale for predicting pressure sore risk. *Nurs Res* **36**(4): 205–10

Black J, Black S (1987) Surgical management of pressure ulcers. *Nurs Clin North America* **22**(2): 429

Bridel J (1993) The aetiology of pressure sores. *J Wound Care* **2**(4): 230–238

Clark M, Fletcher J (1999) Production selection *Journal of Wound Care Mattresses and Beds Resource File.* J Wound Care in association with Huntleigh Healthcare Ltd

David JA, Chapman RG, Chapman EJ (1983) *An Investigation of Current Methods Used in Nursing Care of Patients with Established Pressure Sores.* Northwick Park Research Unit, Harrow

Dealey C (1997) *Managing Pressure Sore Prevention.* Quay Books, Mark Allen Publishing Ltd, Salisbury

Department of Health (1991) *The Health of the Nation.* HMSO, London

Department of Health (2001) *The Essence of Care: Patient focused benchmarking for health care practitioners.* The Stationery Office, London

Department of Health, National Health Service Executive (1998) *Using Electronic Records in Hospital: Legal requirements and good practice.* HSC 1998/153, The Stationery Office, London

Dyson R (1978) Bedsores – the injuries hospital staff inflict on patients. *Nurs Mirror* **146**(24): 30–32

Ek AC, Gustavsson G, Lewis DH (1985) The local skin blood flow in areas at risk of pressure sores treated with massage. *Scand J Rehab Med* **17**(2): 81–6

European Pressure Ulcer Advisory Panel (1998a) *Pressure Ulcer Prevention Guidelines.* www.epuap.org

European Pressure Ulcer Advisory Panel (1998b) *Pressure Ulcer Treatment Guidelines.* www.epuap.org

Fletcher J (1996) Types of pressure-relieving equipment available: 1. *Br J Nurs* **5**(11): 694–701

Hall P (1983) Prophylactic use of Opsite on pressure areas. *Nurs Focus*: January/February

Hampton S (1998) Film subjects win the day. *Nurs Times* **94**(24): 80–2

Health and Safety Executive (1992) *Manual Handling Operations Regulations.* HMSO, London

Health Service Commissioner (2000) The Full Report of Selected Cases, Second Report Session 1999–2000. The Stationery Office, London. www.ombudsman.org.uk

Health Service Commissioner (2001) *The Health Service Commissioner Investigations Completed December 2000–March 2001, Part I, Summaries of investigations completed.* The Stationery Office, London. www.ombudsman.org.uk

Hitch S (1995) NHS Executive strategy for major clinical guidelines — prevention and management of pressure sores — a literature search. *J Tissue Viabil* **5**(4): 111–4

Lennard-Jones JE (1992) *A Positive Approach to Nutrition as a Treatment.* King's Fund Centre, London

Maryon-Davis A, Bristow A (1999) *Managing Nutrition in Hospital: A recipe for quality.* The Nuffield Trust for Research and Policy Studies in Hospital, London

National Audit Commission (1995) *United They Stand: Coordinating care for elderly patients with hip fracture.* The Stationery Office, London

National Institute for Clinical Excellence (2001) *Pressure ulcer risk assessment and prevention.* Inherited Clinical Guideline B. NICE, London: www.nice.org.uk

Newton H, Trudgian J, Gould D (2000) Expanding tissue viability practice through telemedicine. *Br J Nurs* **9**(19): 42–8

Norton D, McClaren R, Exton-Smith AN (1962) *An investigation of Geriatric Nursing Problems in Hospitals.* National Cooperation of the Care of Older People, London

O'Dea K (1993) Prevalence of pressure damage in hospital patients in the UK. *J Wound Care* **2**(4): 221–5

Preston K (1988) Positioning for comfort and pressure relief: the thirty degree alternative. *Care Sci Pract* **6**(4): 116–9

Reid J, Morison M (1994) Towards a consensus classification of pressure sores. *J Wound Care* **3**(3): 157–60

Stacey v *Central Sheffield University Hospital NHS Trust* [2000] The Personal and Medical Injuries Law Letter, November 2000: 6

Tingle J (1997) Pressure sores: counting the legal cost of nursing neglect. *Br J Nurs* **6**(13): 757–8

Torrance C (1983) *Pressure Sores: Aetiology, Treatment and Prevention.* Croom Helm, London

Turner TD (1982) Which dressing and why? *Nurs Times* **78**(Suppl 29): 1–3

United Kingdom Central Council for Nursing, Midwifery and Health Visiting (1992a) *Code of Professional Conduct for the Nurse, Midwife and Health Visitor.* UKCC, London

United Kingdom Central Council for Nursing, Midwifery and Health Visiting (1992b) *The Scope of Professional Practice*. UKCC, London

United Kingdom Central Council for Nursing, Midwifery and Health Visiting (1998) *Guidelines for Records and Record Keeping*. UKCC, London

Waterlow J (1985) Pressure sores: a risk assessment card. *Nurs Times* **81**(48): 49–55

Young J (1992) The use of specialized beds and mattresses. *J Tissue Viabil* **2**(3): 79–81